Eleanor Hannon Judah
Rev. Michael Bryant
Editors

Criminal Justice: Retribution vs. Restoration

Criminal Justice: Retribution vs. Restoration has been co-published simultaneously as *Journal of Religion & Spirituality in Social Work: Social Thought,* Volume 23, Numbers 1/2 2004.

Pre-publication
REVIEWS,
COMMENTARIES,
EVALUATIONS . . .

"The authors make an important contribution to the public policy debate on crime, victimization, and the growing international field of restorative justice. Each chapter provides a much-needed critical examination of issues that policymakers all too frequently avoid ever addressing."

Mark Umbreit, PhD
Professor and Director, Center for Restorative Justice & Peacemaking, University of Minnesota School of Social Work

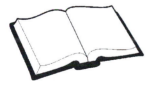

D0222950

More Pre-publication
REVIEWS, COMMENTARIES, EVALUATIONS . . .

"**T**IMELY AND NECESSARY. . . . Of interest to students of social, economic, and behavioral sciences, philosophy, theology, and cultural history, as well as to the general public. As a student and teacher of social policy, social justice, and human development, I find this book thought provoking and I WILL RECOMMEND IT TO MY STUDENTS."

David G. Gil, DSW
Professor of Social Policy
Heller School for Social Policy
and Management, Brandeis
University

"**A**N EXCELLENT RESOURCE for social work educators teaching in the areas of human behavior, policy, and spirituality. . . . I am excited about being able to use this book in my classes and research. Now maybe my students will see that social work education is relevant to work in the criminal justice field and that the principles of restorative justice can serve as the bridge between social work and corrections."

Katherine van Wormer, PhD, MSSW
Professor of Social Work
College of Social & Behavioral Sciences
University of Northern Iowa

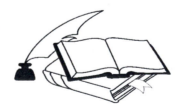

The Haworth Social Work Practice Press
The Haworth Pastoral Press
Imprints of The Haworth Press, Inc.

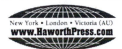

New York • London • Victoria (AU)
www.HaworthPress.com

Criminal Justice: Retribution vs. Restoration

Criminal Justice: Retribution vs. Restoration has been co-published simultaneously as *Journal of Religion & Spirituality in Social Work: Social Thought,* Volume 23, Numbers 1/2 2004.

The *Journal of Religion & Spirituality in Social Work* Monographic "Separates"

Below is a list of "separates," which in serials librarianship means a special issue simultaneously published as a special journal issue or double-issue *and* as a "separate" hardbound monograph. (This is a format which we also call a "DocuSerial.")

"Separates" are published because specialized libraries or professionals may wish to purchase a specific thematic issue by itself in a format which can be separately cataloged and shelved, as opposed to purchasing the journal on an on-going basis. Faculty members may also more easily consider a "separate" for classroom adoption.

"Separates" are carefully classified separately with the major book jobbers so that the journal tie-in can be noted on new book order slips to avoid duplicate purchasing.

You may wish to visit Haworth's website at . . .

http://www.HaworthPress.com

. . . to search our online catalog for complete tables of contents of these separates and related publications.

You may also call 1-800-HAWORTH (outside US/Canada: 607-722-5857), or Fax 1-800-895-0582 (outside US/Canada: 607-771-0012), or e-mail at:

docdelivery@haworthpress.com

Criminal Justice: Retribution vs. Restoration, edited by Eleanor Hannon Judah, DSW, ACSW, and Rev. Michael Bryant, PhD (Vol. 23, No. 1/2, 2004). *"Timely and necessary. . . . Of interest to students of social, economic, and behavioral sciences, philosophy, theology, and cultural history, as well as to the general public. As a student and teacher of social policy, social justice, and human development, I find this book thought provoking and I will recommend it to my students."* (David G. Gil, DSW, Professor of Social Policy, Heller School for Social Policy and Management, Brandeis University)

Practicing Social Justice, * edited by John J. Stretch, PhD, MBA, ACSW, LCSW, Ellen M. Burkemper, PhD, LCSW, MFT, William J. Hutchison, PhD, and Jan Wilson, ACSW, LCSW (Vol. 22, No. 2/3, 2003). *"I highly recommend this important edited work to practitioners, academics, and students majoring in the human services and related fields. . . . Fills an important void in the area of social justice and related issues. . . . Offers a detailed analysis of numerous social justice issues."* (John T. Pardeck, PhD, LCSW, Editor, Journal of Social Work in Disability and Rehabilitation)

Issues in Global Aging, * edited by Frederick L. Ahearn, Jr., DSW (Vol. 20, No. 3/4, 2001). *"Fine scholarship . . . very useful. Ahearn has assembled a fine cohort of experts on aging who address various issues. The first section approaches them from the western industrial model perspective, but also provides an example of an Islamic traditional approach. The second section deals less with formal religiosity than with issues of spiritual transcendence in older persons. A balanced portrait of the aged as people rather than statistics."* (Charles Guzzetta, EdD, Professor, Hunter College, City University of New York)

Transpersonal Perspectives on Spirituality in Social Work, * edited by Edward R. Canda, PhD, and Elizabeth D. Smith, DSW (Vol. 20, No. 1/2, 2001). *"Comprehensive . . . provides theoretical and practice-oriented studies on the emerging field of Transpersonal social work. The writing is both scholarly and relevant to practice. Of interest to scholars, practitioners, and students alike."* (John R. Graham, PhD, RSW, Associate Professor, Faculty of Social Work, University of Calgary, Alberta, Canada)

Raising Our Children Out of Poverty, * edited by John J. Stretch, PhD, Maria Bartlett, PhD, William J. Hutchison, PhD, Susan A. Taylor, PhD, and Jan Wilson, MSW (Vol. 19, No. 2, 1999). *This book shows what can be done at the national and local community levels to raise children out of poverty by strengthening families, communities, and social services.*

Postmodernism, Religion and the Future of Social Work, * edited by Roland G. Meinert, PhD, John T. Pardeck, PhD, and John W. Murphy, PhD (Vol. 18, No. 3, 1998). *"Critically important for social work as it attempts to effectively respond to its increasingly complex roles and demands. . . .*

A book worth owning and studying." (John M. Herrick, PhD, Acting Director, School of Social Work, Michigan State University, East Lansing, Michigan)

Spirituality in Social Work: New Directions,* edited by Edward R. Canda, PhD (Vol. 18, No. 2, 1998). *"Provides interesting insights and references for those who seek to develop curricula responsive to the spiritual challenges confronting our profession and the populations we serve."* (Au-Deane S. Cowley, PhD, Associate Dean, Graduate School of Social Work, University of Utah, Salt Lake City)

*Published under the title *Social Thought: Journal of Religion in the Social Services*

Published by

The Haworth Social Work Practice Press, 10 Alice Street, Binghamton, NY 13904-1580 USA

The Haworth Social Work Practice Press is an imprint of The Haworth Press, Inc., 10 Alice Street, Binghamton, NY 13904-1580 USA.

Criminal Justice: Retribution vs. Restoration has been co-published simultaneously as *Journal of Religion & Spirituality in Social Work,* Volume 23, Numbers 1/2 2004.

The development, preparation, and publication of this work has been undertaken with great care. However, the publisher, employees, editors, and agents of The Haworth Press and all imprints of The Haworth Press, Inc., including The Haworth Medical Press® and The Pharmaceutical Products Press®, are not responsible for any errors contained herein or for consequences that may ensue from use of materials or information contained in this work. Opinions expressed by the author(s) are not necessarily those of The Haworth Press, Inc. With regard to case studies, identities and circumstances of individuals discussed herein have been changed to protect confidentiality. Any resemblence to actual persons, living or dead, is entirely coincidental.

Cover design by Brooke R. Stiles

Library of Congress Cataloging-in-Publication Data

Criminal justice : retribution vs. restoration / Eleanor Hannon Judah, Michael Bryant, editors.
     p. cm.
     "Co-published simultaneously as Journal of Religion & Spirituality in Social Work, Volume 23, Numbers 1/2 2004."
     Includes bibliographical references and index.
     ISBN 0-7890-0061-X (cloth : alk. paper) – ISBN 0-7890-0081-4 (pbk. : alk. paper)
     1. Criminal justice, Administration of–United States 2. Punishment–United States. 3. Criminals–Rehabilitation–United States. I. Judah, Eleanor Hannon. II. Bryant, Michael, Rev. III. Journal of religion & spirituality in social work.
HV9950.C74322 2004
364.973–dc22
                                      2003023849

Criminal Justice: Retribution vs. Restoration

Eleanor Hannon Judah
Rev. Michael Bryant
Editors

Criminal Justice: Retribution vs. Restoration has been co-published simultaneously as *Journal of Religion & Spirituality in Social Work: Social Thought,* Volume 23, Numbers 1/2 2004.

The Haworth Social Work Practice Press
The Haworth Pastoral Press
Imprints of The Haworth Press, Inc.

New York • London • Victoria (AU)
www.HaworthPress.com

Indexing, Abstracting & Website/Internet Coverage

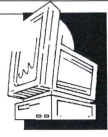

This section provides you with a list of major indexing & abstracting services. That is to say, each service began covering this periodical during the year noted in the right column. Most Websites which are listed below have indicated that they will either post, disseminate, compile, archive, cite or alert their own Website users with research-based content from this work. (This list is as current as the copyright date of this publication.)

Abstracting, Website/Indexing Coverage . . . . Year When Coverage Began

- *Applied Social Sciences Index & Abstracts (ASSIA)*
  (Online: ASSI via Data-Star) (CDRom: ASSIA Plus)
  <http://www.csa.com> **1998**

- *CareData: The supporting social care management and*
  practice <http://www.elsc.org.uk/caredata/caredata.htm> **1995**

- *Catholic Periodical & Literature Index (CPLI), The* **2001**

- *CINAHL (Cumulative Index to Nursing & Allied Health*
  Literature), in print, EBSCO, and SilverPlatter,
  Data-Star, and PaperChase <http://www.cinahl.com> **2000**

- *CNPIEC Reference Guide: Chinese National Directory*
  of Foreign Periodicals **1995**

- *EAP Abstracts Plus* **2000**

- *Family Index Database <http://www.familyscholar.com>* **2003**

- *Family & Society Studies Worldwide <http://www.nisc.com>* **2000**

- *FRANCIS. INIST/CNRS <http://www.inist.fr>* **1999**

- *Guide to Social Science and Religion in Periodical Literature* **1995**

(continued)

*Special Bibliographic Notes related to special journal issues
(separates) and indexing/abstracting:*

- indexing/abstracting services in this list will also cover material in any "separate" that is co-published simultaneously with Haworth's special thematic journal issue or DocuSerial. Indexing/abstracting usually covers material at the article/chapter level.
- monographic co-editions are intended for either non-subscribers or libraries which intend to purchase a second copy for their circulating collections.
- monographic co-editions are reported to all jobbers/wholesalers/approval plans. The source journal is listed as the "series" to assist the prevention of duplicate purchasing in the same manner utilized for books-in-series.
- to facilitate user/access services all indexing/abstracting services are encouraged to utilize the co-indexing entry note indicated at the bottom of the first page of each article/chapter/contribution.
- this is intended to assist a library user of any reference tool (whether print, electronic, online, or CD-ROM) to locate the monographic version if the library has purchased this version but not a subscription to the source journal.
- individual articles/chapters in any Haworth publication are also available through the Haworth Document Delivery Service (HDDS).
- individual articles/chapters in any Haworth publication are also available through the Haworth Document Delivery Service (HDDS).

Criminal Justice: Retribution vs. Restoration

CONTENTS

ABOUT THE EDITORS

Eleanor Hannon Judah, DSW, ACSW, is the Book Review Editor and former Editor of *Social Thought*. She is a retired Associate Professor of the National Catholic School of Social Service at The Catholic University of America in Washington, DC. Since 1998, as Associate Chaplain at the District of Columbia Detention Facility, she has given direct service weekly to inmates at the DC Jail. Dr. Judah's social work practice experience in Pittsburgh, Washington, Hartford, and Birmingham, England, includes direct practice, supervision, field instruction, and consultation, primarily in services to families and child placement. As a Fulbright Scholar at the University of Birmingham, she researched policy and services to homeless and multi-problem families in a welfare state.

Dr. Judah's professional publications appear in *Social Casework,* the *Journal of Social Work Education, Social Thought, Charities USA, and Social Work* (British). These publications focused on student acculturation and value change in professional education for social work, the role of hope in the helping process, spirituality, and long-range strategic planning for social agencies.

Rev. Michael Bryant, PhD, holds master's degrees in theology and psychology and a PhD in pastoral counseling. He is a licensed mental health therapist, a supervisor in clinical pastoral education, and a former Adjunct Professor at The Catholic University of America, the DeSales School of Theology, and the Washington Theological Union. He is currently in his 24th year as chaplain at the District of Columbia Detention Facility.

Reverend Bryant is the author of numerous articles addressing the Church and prison reform issues, and is a contributing author to *Who Is the Prisoner?* He was involved in the development of the recently released national statement from the United States Catholic Bishops, "Responsibility, Rehabilitation, and Restoration." He is past Chair of the National Convocation of Jail and Prison Ministry–an organization that advocates prison reform and opposition to the death penalty. Prior service includes 12 years in parish ministries as an associate pastor and later as pastor. Reverend Bryant regularly addresses national and local audiences on criminal justice reform.

INTRODUCTION

Rethinking Criminal Justice:
Retribution vs. Restoration

Eleanor Hannon Judah
Rev. Michael Bryant

This special volume emerged out of the collective experience of almost thirty years ministering as chaplains in the city jail in Washington, DC, and years of social work, and after listening to the tragic stories of thousands of confined men and women and others. Observing the justice system at work and its effects on the lives of so many broken people and devastated families and communities leads us to believe that there must be a better way of doing justice in our society not only for offenders, but for victims and the community as well. We believe *restorative justice* offers such hope.

Our present criminal justice philosophy is based on the concept of *retribution*, that is, "something given or demanded in repayment, especially punishment" (Webster II, 1995), the punishment most often inflicted through imprisonment. This system has failed. But what is meant by *restorative justice*? It is an entirely different way of approaching crime. "It asks firstly, not how do we punish, but how do we repair the damage done? As a process it offers victims, offenders, and the community positive ways

[Haworth co-indexing entry note]: "Rethinking Criminal Justice: Retribution vs. Restoration." Judah, Eleanor Hannon, and Rev. Michael Bryant. Co-published simultaneously in *Journal of Religion & Spirituality in Social Work* (The Haworth Social Work Practice Press, an imprint of The Haworth Press, Inc.) Vol. 23, No. 1/2, 2004, pp. 1-6; and: *Criminal Justice: Retribution vs. Restoration* (ed: Eleanor Hannon Judah, and Rev. Michael Bryant) The Haworth Social Work Practice Press, an imprint of The Haworth Press, Inc., 2004, pp. 1-6. Single or multiple copies of this article are available for a fee from The Haworth Document Delivery Service [1-800- HAWORTH, 9:00 a.m. - 5:00 p.m. (EST). E-mail address: docdelivery@haworthpress.com].

http://www.haworthpress.com/web/JRSSW
Digital Object Identifier: 10.1300/J377v23n01_01

forward that help heal the trauma of crime and reduce reoffending" (Consedine & Bowen, 1999).

WHY CHANGE?

In many ways our criminal justice system is closed to the public. Even though courts are open, few citizens involve themselves in court proceedings. Even fewer citizens have an opportunity to observe life behind bars. Establishing policies and legislative action affecting the justice system is left to state and federal legislators who frequently make "get tough" decisions that win them public favor and votes. The media tend to provide the public with the sensational provocative stories that swirl around heinous crimes and punishment, but most often fail to address systemic issues underlying the failure of the justice system. Both legislators and the media provide the public with little appreciation of the raw reality of the system and how it impacts those caught up in it.

Like other professionals, social workers and pastoral counselors know the struggles of families who are victims of crime or have a family member incarcerated, but are often unaware of the magnitude of the effect the justice system has on their clients, thus failing to advocate for reappraisal and change of the system.

Crime victims are usually left to fend for themselves in a system of justice that cares little for them as individuals who have been violated. They are usually either ignored or used by the prosecution as witnesses and then dismissed without recourse of counseling or remuneration.

The proliferation of drugs and the unbridled use of lethal weapons are a deadly reality for millions of Americans. In urban environments a concentration of people of color who are often poor and poorly educated are prime candidates for the justice system, as are the addicted, mentally ill and jobless.

The criminal justice system is clearly in crisis. Currently, two million people in the United States are imprisoned; another 4.7 million are on parole or probation. One consequence of our race to incarcerate is the six hundred thousand men and women who will be released from prison each year for the foreseeable future (Bureau of Justice Statistics, 2002). And an astounding nine million will cycle back to the community from local jails (Bureau of Justice Statistics, 2002). The criminal justice system is clearly in crisis.

If the enormous toll in human suffering and social disintegration are not convincing enough, perhaps the staggering economic costs of maintaining such a system of mass incarceration in this era of belt tightening may attract and persuade skeptics that "compassionate conservatism" may demand a more humane (and cheaper) approach.

This collection both documents some of the failures of our present system and offers a better way to think about and do criminal justice, moving beyond the confines of the blame and punishment of retributive justice. Conceived and resting on Biblical concepts of restoration, healing, forgiveness, reconciliation and responsibility, it is intrinsically more compatible and, it is thought, more attractive to the basic philosophy, ethics and values of the readers than the punitive retribution model now in force.

This work is unique in the variety of perspectives offered, and in the fact that all contributors are currently actively involved in some capacity in criminal justice as scholars, researchers, advocates, restorative practioners, social workers and founders of programs, as well as a victim and an incarcerated man. All see an urgent need for "rethinking criminal justice."

THE BROKEN SYSTEM

Mauer and Coyle set the stage with an overview of our present policy of mass incarceration and its enormous social cost. Braman follows with an up-close and poignant view of the devastation to family networks caused by repeated incarceration of an addicted parent. Sterling connects public policy and racial issues impacting on the use of criminalization of and imprisonment for drug use and the targeting of racial minorities for arrest. In contrast, Johnson presents a glimpse of what is possible with a restorative approach, even within our present punitive system. Still imprisoned after 27 years for a sex assault, he writes of the profound effect of forgiveness in a long delayed meeting with his victim and having the opportunity to take responsibility for his offence, to express his sorrow to her, and to receive her forgiveness.

ANOTHER WAY

On a hope filled note, Van Ness, in "Justice that Restores," then lays out the basics of another way, *restorative justice*, an approach that is personal, not impersonal, designed to heal, not just to blame and punish. In Misleh and Hanneman, we learn of the embrace of restorative justice by communities of faith, many of who have already embarked on programs of promotion, education and service. Pranis, a restorative justice practioner and planner for a state corrections system, addresses the questions of what restorative justice looks like and its efficacy. She describes practices of restorative justice in criminal justice and other contexts as well as its challenges and limitations. Jaeger Lane, mother of a murdered child, then tells of her own journey from fury to forgiveness of the man who abducted and killed her young daughter.

GETTING THERE

Travis speaks to the consequences to communities of extremely high incarceration rates, which in time vitiate morale and resiliency and impede the capacity to function as a community, and suggests a role for community engagement in reducing the current reliance on incarceration. Galbraith spells out the unique characteristics of women inmates and, using the program she founded, offers a model for empowering and supporting women while incarcerated and upon return to the community. Reamer discusses the devolution of the social work profession's early involvement in criminal justice, and offers suggestions for reintegration of social work and criminal justice in ways that reflect its unique values and mission. Finally, the Sullivans, founders of a national criminal justice grass roots advocacy organization, recount the 30-year saga of two determined advocates for criminal justice reform. The wins and the losses, the epiphanies and false starts are recounted, but, in the end, the conclusion: "The struggle is its own reward."

QUO VADIS?

The philosophy/process/practice of restorative justice is emerging in many settings from state prisons systems to small community groups in response to a growing recognition that a criminal justice system that has abandoned rehabilitation for punishment at great economic and social costs, and has staggering recidivism rates, has largely failed. In contrast to other enterprises, the growth of our incarceration corrections enterprise thrives on its own failure to "correct." The poorer the job, the better the growth. In a tragic paradox, *its failure is its success.*

Public social policy change comes when a vision of a better way of confronting problems is in view, a "paradigm shift." Only then can problems be redefined and novel solutions proposed. Restorative justice practice offers glimpses of just such a vision, even as it is in the process of its own development as a way to do justice. It attracts with its humane and hope filled, new yet ancient philosophy and vision of true justice based on restoration, restitution, forgiveness, and reconciliation. As in the best social work practice, it takes a holistic, system-wide view of the social situation, includes all players in solutions, affirms the dignity, worth and uniqueness of every human involved and their capacity for growth and change; its dynamic is strength based and empowering. It is even inspiring, for *there is nothing so powerful as an idea whose time has come.*

CONCLUSION

The profession of social work, having backed away from its early and distinguished involvement in criminal justice as the more punitive approach strengthened, now has a unique opportunity to become a part of an approach that is entirely compatible with the profession's philosophy, ethics and values. Social workers can not only contribute their skills in the many aspects of the practice of restorative justice, but importantly, can help to define policy issues and strategies, propose solutions in human terms, conduct research on emerging policy and practice and advocate for change.

Pastoral counselors and others in faith-based communities share many of the ethics and values of social workers. Churches, mosques, synagogues and other groups too are often sleeping giants in the area of criminal justice reform. Agents of reconciliation and healing, faith communities in partnership with government may have increasing opportunities to ease the pain of victims, give support to men and women returning from prison and help to reestablish peace and order in communities. Further, with new knowledge of restorative approaches to criminal justice, faith communities are increasingly recognizing their own moral authority and obligation to challenge existing public policy and to work toward restoration and healing to all who are touched by crime.

REFERENCES

Bureau of Justice Statistics (2001). *Prison statistic: Probation and parole statistics: Recent trends*. Washington DC: U.S. Department of Justice.

Consedine, J. & Bowen H. (Eds.) (1999). *Restorative justice: Contemporary themes and practice*. Lyttleton, New Zealand: Ploughshares Publications.

Personal Communication with Alan Beck, Bureau of Justice Statistics, February 13, 2003.

Webster's II New College Dictionary (1995). Boston/New York: Houghton Mifflin Co.

The Social Cost
of America's Race to Incarcerate

Marc Mauer
Michael Coyle

SUMMARY. Over the past three decades, the United States has been engaged in an unprecedented expansion of its prison system, with the national inmate population rising from just over 300,000 in 1972 to nearly two million today. Much of this increase has been related to an overreliance on the criminal justice system as a means of responding to social problems and, in particular, to the expansion of harsh sentencing policies. There is little evidence that these policies have had any substantial impact on crime, but they have been increasingly harmful to family and neighborhood stability in low-income communities of color. *[Article copies available for a fee from The Haworth Document Delivery Service: 1-800-HAWORTH. E-mail address: <docdelivery@haworthpress.com> Website: <http://www.HaworthPress.com> © 2004 by The Haworth Press, Inc. All rights reserved.]*

Marc Mauer, MSW, is Assistant Director of The Sentencing Project and the author of *Race to Incarcerate* (The New Press) and the editor, with Meda Chesney-Lind, of *Invisible Punishment: The Collateral Consequences of Mass Imprisonment* (The New Press). Address correspondence to: The Sentencing Project, 514 10th Street NW, Suite 1000, Washington, DC 20004 (E-mail: mauer@sentencingproject.org).

Michael Coyle, MTS, is a PhD student in Justice Studies at Arizona State University. His research interests include class, ethnicity, and race in incarceration, prisoners' human rights, and alternatives to incarceration. Address correspondence to: School of Justice Studies, Arizona State University, P.O. Box 870403, Tempe, AZ 85287-0403 (E-mail: Michael.Coyle@asu.edu).

[Haworth co-indexing entry note]: "The Social Cost of America's Race to Incarcerate." Mauer, Marc, and Michael Coyle. Co-published simultaneously in *Journal of Religion & Spirituality in Social Work* (The Haworth Social Work Practice Press, an imprint of The Haworth Press, Inc.) Vol. 23, No. 1/2, 2004, pp. 7-25; and: *Criminal Justice: Retribution vs. Restoration* (ed: Eleanor Hannon Judah, and Rev. Michael Bryant) The Haworth Social Work Practice Press, an imprint of The Haworth Press, Inc., 2004, pp. 7-25. Single or multiple copies of this article are available for a fee from The Haworth Document Delivery Service [1-800-HAWORTH, 9:00 a.m. - 5:00 p.m. (EST). E-mail address: docdelivery@haworthpress.com].

http://www.haworthpress.com/web/JRSSW
© 2004 by The Haworth Press, Inc. All rights reserved.
Digital Object Identifier: 10.1300/J377v23n01_02

KEYWORDS. Incarceration, sentencing, racial disparity, crime control

COMPARING SOCIAL PROBLEMS AND APPROACHES

In the mid-1980s the United States was wracked by a profound health crisis that was both unique and frightening. As the nation began to learn of the rapid spread of the HIV virus, public attention and significant federal resources focused on discovering the source of the virus and on developing the means of effectively responding to it. Fifteen years later, there has been a tremendous toll in human lives and suffering, but important progress has been made as well. HIV/AIDS education and prevention curricula are now commonplace in a vast array of school and community settings, and the rapid development of new drug therapies has served to enable many with the disease to continue to lead productive lives.

Coinciding with the rapid spread of HIV/AIDS in the mid-1980s was another epidemic that also brought great tragedy and suffering. This epidemic was one of violence associated with the introduction and spread of crack cocaine, initially in urban areas and then spreading to other communities. As teenagers and others in many neighborhoods armed themselves with lethal weapons to protect their drug "turf," murder rates spiked sharply in the second half of the 1980s, particularly among African American males.

The reaction to crack cocaine and the violence that initially came with it among policymakers was swift and certain. However, instead of a calculated study of the problem, and an investment in education and prevention, as with the HIV/AIDS epidemic, a host of harsh sentencing laws were adopted. The most notorious of these were the federal provisions mandating a five-year prison sentence for possession of five grams of crack–the weight of two pennies. Along with this came a wave of new prison construction and an incarceration binge that has sent the nation's inmate population soaring from 500,000 in 1980 to nearly two million today (BJS, 1981, 1991, 2002). This prison building frenzy served to accelerate the prison expansion that had begun in the 1970s, and has led to the United States now having attained the dubious distinction of maintaining the world's highest rate of incarceration (Facts About Prisons and Prisoners, 2002).

The two epidemics of the 1980s offer a useful opportunity to contrast the development of public policy. Imagine for a moment that in response to the HIV/AIDS epidemic national leaders had instead proclaimed a policy of massive hospital construction to cope with the sick and dying population. Ever larger institutions would have been built through infusions of federal and state funds, even as the death toll continued to mount. Instead of budget increases for federal research on the disease or for investigating personal lifestyle changes to reduce the chances of contagion, all investments would have gone toward increasing bed space.

The notion of confronting a health crisis by building hospitals is ludicrous, of course, but in our national imagination the idea of building prisons to confront a crime problem has become the policy of choice. How, then, did we come to view these two crises in such different terms?

To be sure, the national response to HIV/AIDS was far from an entirely compassionate one from the beginning. As AIDS was initially perceived as a "gay disease," some Americans viewed it as a deserved punishment for "immoral" behavior. Political leaders in many cases acted only reluctantly after massive mobilizations by the gay community and public health advocates. But in no instance did the notion of hospital construction as a "solution" ever enter anyone's mind.

Why we view disease and crime in such strikingly different terms is complex, but several factors can help us understand the roots of this dichotomy. On the one hand, in the case of HIV/AIDS, many Americans quickly realized that a sexually transmitted disease was a threat not just to others but also to themselves and their loved ones. As such, rhetoric of "blaming the victim" was hardly an approach to bring comfort in most homes. Furthermore, as more "celebrity" victims emerged, the public face of the disease changed and a more compassionate and public health-oriented response emerged.

In the HIV/AIDS epidemic the initial public perception was to view it as a gay disease. In time, however, this gave way to an understanding of HIV/AIDS as a national epidemic with large medical, but also social, consequences. Eventually, HIV/AIDS was grasped as a problem, which the whole community would have to engage if it was to be successfully battled. Thus, the public perception was transformed from one of a "gay disease" to annual fundraising walks, massive billboard campaigns, an education movement for safe sex, and much more.

In examining the crime problem though, the public perception of the "criminal" became dominant, and it remains dominant, in determining the direction of policy. Just as various waves of European immigrants were viewed as the source of the crime problem in the early years of the twentieth century, so too have African Americans and Hispanics now become the public image of the "criminal." As this perception has remained pervasive, the policy response has been one that emphasizes punishment and incarceration over an approach that engages the nation in a search for causes and cures.

RESPONSE TO CRIME: PUNISHMENT AND INCARCERATION AS POLICY

In the United States, despite relative prosperity and abundant wealth in world terms, we have now reached the remarkable total of two million Americans behind bars in the nation's prisons and jails. The figure is dramatic enough (more than the entire population of 15 states, for example), but it gains even more significance when we examine it in historical and global terms. In this regard, the scale of increase over the past thirty years is unprecedented in both American history and that of any democratic nation since the birth of the penitentiary. While for fifty years the national inmate population remained steady, in 1972 it began a rapid and continuous rise that has gone unabated for three decades.

An international perspective reveals that incarceration is used to a far greater extent in the U.S. than in any other industrialized nation. Currently, the U.S. locks up its citizens at 6-10 times the rate of most comparable nations (Mauer, 1999). In the year 2000 the U.S. achieved the dubious distinction of outpacing its arch rival Russia in what might be called the "imprisonment race" to regain the world lead in per capita incarceration. As of 2001 the rate of incarceration in the U.S. was 690 inmates per 100,000 population as compared to Russia's 676 inmates per 100,000 population. This resulted from the combined impact of continuing punitiveness in the U.S. along with a Russian amnesty of more than 100,000 prisoners designed to reduce the horrendous overcrowding and disease that pervades its prison system (Facts About Prisons and Prisoners, 2002).

The international comparison of scales of incarceration is telling, but it does not inform us as to why some nations employ prisons more than others. At a basic level, there are two factors that can contribute to such an outcome: crime rates and criminal justice policies. All things being equal, a nation with a high rate of crime or with harsh sentencing policies might be expected to have a high rate of imprisonment. Without dissecting these issues in great detail here, we know that both of these factors play a role in understanding the use of mass imprisonment in the U.S.

While there is little evidence to suggest that rates of property crime are considerably different in the U.S. than in other industrialized nations, rates of violent crime are substantially greater. Even with a substantial decline in homicide during the 1990s, U.S. homicide rates are still almost five times those of most European nations (Lynch, 1995). Much, though not all, of this disparity relates to the proliferation of firearms in the U.S. and the greater frequency in which a dispute or assault can turn into a murder. Also, while comparative data are limited, there is evidence that property and drug offenders in the U.S. receive longer prison sentences than similar offenders in other nations (Lynch, 1995). Further, as a result of the twenty-year "war on drugs," drug offenders account for a substantial portion of the prison population increase–now nearly one of every four inmates. Overall, the number of drug offenders has increased ten-fold from about 40,000 in 1980 to more than 450,000 today (BJS, 1996, 2000a). Added to this is the increasingly punitive nature of American attitudes toward juveniles, which is in sharp contrast with other democratic nations, most of which have little understanding how a crime committed by a 12-year-old can result in a sentence of life without parole.

Some observers suggest that mass imprisonment is merely an unfortunate, but necessary, outcome of a nation with a propensity for crime. Such commentary is rare among those demographic groups most subject to the incarceration binge, but it is also odd in the degree to which it suggests an implicit acceptance of both high rates of imprisonment *and* high rates of crime in the world's wealthiest society.

Even to the extent that crime explains some of the propensity for prison building and massive incarceration, this tells us little about the wisdom or efficacy of such a policy. The issue is most clear in regard to drug offenses, particularly given the ten-fold increase in incarcerated drug offenders from 1980 to today. At an annual cost of imprisonment of $20,000 per prisoner and much documentation that most drug offenders are not the kingpins of the trade, this is a social policy that defies all logic. It also stands in direct opposition to most research evidence regarding effective approaches to the reduction of substance abuse.

In the absence of a clearly thought out *policy on the use of imprisonment*, what exist are *policies for imprisonment*. As in the crack cocaine sentencing legislation, there is an assumption that increased imprisonment leads to decreased crime. In fact, many of the sentencing policies put into effect in the last few decades, despite their stated intent to curb crime, have had questionable effects on crime reduction and have been strongly critiqued for creating new sets of problems (economic ruin in inner cities) or exacerbating already existing ones (tense class and race relations).

Two such initiatives have been mandatory sentencing and three-strikes laws. In mandatory sentencing legislators created law that requires a mandatory specified prison term for a particular offense. The result is the removal of the traditional discretion of judges to determine what sentence should be imposed on an offender based on a consideration of the circumstances of the crime and other relevant factors. Since the early 1990s a growing body of scholarly research has been asking whether mandatory minimum sentencing statutes have been successful in achieving their purposes. A 1994 study by the Federal Judicial Center summarized the research to date and suggested that mandatory minimums compromise the basic fairness and integrity of the federal criminal justice system (Vincent & Hofer, 1994).

Chief Justice William Rehnquist (1993) has described mandatory sentencing as statutes that are "perhaps a good example of the law of unintended consequences." Certainly, there are those who assert that mandatory minimum sentences are worth the price, and who believe that the negative effects are overstated, and that mandatory minimums serve important symbolic functions and have a broad deterrent effect—or will have a deterrent effect as public knowledge of legislative resolve to punish crime severely increases. But three decades later such fruits have not materialized. In fact, there is now substantial evidence that mandatory minimums result every year in the lengthy incarceration of thousands of low-level offenders who could be effectively sentenced to shorter periods of time or community supervision at annual savings of several hundred million dollars (USSC, 2002). There is also evidence that mandatory minimums do not narrowly target violent criminals or major drug traffickers, as they were purportedly designed to do (USSC, 2002).

Another significant policy trend of the early 1990s was three-strikes legislation. By 1995 twenty-three states and the federal government had adopted some type of "three strikes and you're out" law with the intent of targeting repeat violent offenders. The state of Washington was the first to do so in 1993, and California soon followed with a considerably broader version. Although subsequently adopted versions of three-strikes law varied among the states, they generally reduced judicial discretion by mandating severe prison sentences for third (and in some instances second) felony convictions.

The "three strikes" bandwagon was set in motion at a time when public fear of crime was at its height. These laws came with extravagant promises of crime reduction that ensured passage in many states. Soon, however, closer examination began to document the law's uneven application and its significant impact on state budgets and prison admissions (Dickey, 1996). It was found that while political rhetoric dominated much of the debate preceding the adoption of these laws, widely speaking they were mostly having a minimal impact (King & Mauer, 2001). Their implementation was found to come at great economic cost, with little demonstrated impact on crime. In California, the state with the most wide-ranging law, a key impact was the imprisonment of less serious offenders to long prison terms just as they were aging out of their "crime prone" years (Dickey & Hollenhorst, 1998). Two-thirds of the offenders affected by the law had been convicted of nonviolent offenses (King & Mauer, 2001). Research also found that prosecutorial discretion and plea-bargaining resulted in very uneven application of the law between different jurisdictions within the state, and that while African-Americans comprised 31% of the total inmates in the state's prisons, they were 37% of offenders convicted under two strikes and 44% of offenders convicted under three strikes.

EFFECTS OF PREVAILING POLICY ON CRIME

Traditionally, the impact of incarceration policies is assessed by asking to what extent incarceration can be demonstrated to have had an impact on crime rates. Assessing this relationship turns out to be more complicated than one might assume because, as with any social science observation, a variety of factors that may affect crime rates are generally occurring simultaneously. However, recent experience provides some guidance.

Over the last few years many policymakers have argued that the success of current incarceration policies can be viewed in the declining crime rates of the 1990s. During the seven-year period 1991-98, for example, the rate of incarceration rose by 47% and crime rates declined by 22%. For some, this appears as a simple cause and effect relationship. However, the relationship turns out to be far more complex. The first complication is the apparently contradictory period just prior to this, from 1984 to 1991. During these seven years, the rate of incarceration also rose substantially, by 65%, but the crime rate also rose by 17% (Gainsborough & Mauer, 2000). Thus, the initial period no more proves that incarceration *causes* crime than the second period illustrates that it *reduces* crime. These contrasting periods do not suggest that incarceration rates have no effect on crime rates, but they should make us cautious about assuming that building and filling prisons will always result in lower crime rates.

While it might seem intuitively obvious that putting more people in prison would reduce crime, in fact there are sound criminological reasons why this is not always the case. Among the most significant factors complicating this relationship is the impact of incarceration on varying types of crime. Prosecuting and imprisoning a serial rapist undoubtedly makes a neighborhood safer. But expanding the prison population by locking up tens of thousands of low-level drug offenders has relatively little impact on crime or drug abuse. One of the reasons for this is that drug sellers, unlike serial rapists, are readily replaceable. As long as a strong demand for illegal drugs exists, new sellers will be easily recruited to the market.

Criminologists differ on the degree to which incarceration can be said to affect crime, but it is fair to say that the prevailing mainstream view in the field is that this relationship is considerably weaker than that promised by the political sponsors of "get tough" policies. Recent scholarship on crime reductions in the 1990s suggests that perhaps 25% of the reduction in violent crime can be attributed to prison building (Spelman, 2000; Rosenfeld, 2000). While such a reduction is quite welcome it fails to explain three-quarters of the crime drop, not to mention the inconsistent results of the late 1980s, which, as illustrated, had the opposite trend. While the "prison-time reduces crime" relationship is subject to debate, it is the near consensus among scholars that fluctuations in crime rates are subject to a host of complex factors other than imprisonment. These factors include individual personality, family dynamics, employment and educational prospects, substance abuse, and many others.

Much of the change in crime rates over the past 15 years can be explained by tracking changes in drug use trends and the economy. As crack cocaine emerged initially in urban areas in the mid-1980s a thriving illicit drug market developed which provided opportunities for young men (and increasingly women) to establish themselves as entrepreneurs. Added to the mix was the ready access to illegal guns, which turned a mini drug epidemic into an outbreak of violence and homicide. For several years, murder rates spiked sharply, particularly among young African American males.

These murder rates, however, shifted with the maturation of the crack market. While lawmakers and the media engaged in the politics of hysteria at the expense of a studied approach to the problem, rates of crime and violence began to drop in the early 1990s as rapidly as they had previously risen. As was true in previous drug epidemics, the period of youthful infatuation with the drug was short lived. Gradually, many young people and their parents came to realize the dangers of crack and turned away from it. In addition, police in some cities began to make more aggressive efforts to track the supply of illegal weapons into neighborhoods. Finally, sadly, many of the most active offenders ended up dead, imprisoned, or having succumbed to AIDS.

Coincident with these changes was an improvement in the overall economic health of the nation. As unemployment rates declined in the 1990s (aided in part by an expanding prison population), more job opportunities opened up, most significantly in the low-wage sector to which many ex-offenders or potential offenders gravitate. The impact of these changes on crime is similarly difficult to gauge, but at least one rigorous analysis estimates that declines in unemployment were responsible for 30% of the decline in crime from 1992 to 1997 (Freeman & Rodgers, 1999).

Even to the extent that incarceration can be correlated with reductions in crime, this does not inform us as to whether this is the only, or most effective, approach to the problem. After all, if half the population were in prison and guarded by the other half, we would no doubt see reduced crime, but we would hardly consider that an effective or humane approach to the problem. In fact, research in a number of disciplines demonstrates that a variety of social investments can produce more significant reductions in certain types of crime than expanded prison construction. For example, a RAND study found that spending on drug treatment would reduce serious crimes fifteen times more effectively than incapacitating offenders through mandatory prison terms (Caulkins et al., 1997).

In sum, prevailing crime policies should prove troubling to all Americans. First, we maintain the odd position of being the wealthiest society in human history while also locking up more of our citizens than any nation of any age. Second, the racial dynamics of these policies are profound—at current rates of imprisonment, 29% of black males born today can expect to go to prison at some point in their lives, as well as 16% of Latino males and 4% of white males (Bonczar & Beck, 1997). Surely these are not trends that should be welcomed, regardless of one's beliefs about the causes of these developments.

EFFECTS OF PREVAILING POLICY ON SOCIETY

While examining the prison-crime relationship is important, it risks obscuring a deeper analysis of the effects of mass imprisonment on society. The effects of a prison experience on the individual inmate and his or her family appear on many levels intuitive. However, at the level of mass incarceration that we have reached today, an analysis of the impact of prison by necessity must go beyond the individual prisoner and explore how these policies affect society broadly.

Not surprisingly, one of the most prominent social impacts of mass imprisonment is how it is unequally borne by minorities. This impact is felt most dramatically in the African American community, which is experiencing astonishing rates of incarceration. Among adult black males, one in 22 is in prison or jail on any given day. In the age group 25-34 the figure reaches one in nine (BJS, 2000b). Comparable figures for black women are lower overall, but have been rising at dramatic rates and outpace the incarceration of white women by a six to one ratio.

While about half of African American prisoners are incarcerated for a violent offense (as is true for all racial/ethnic groups), the explosion of drug sentences has affected their wider communities profoundly. Though government surveys document that African Americans represent 13% of monthly drug users, they currently constitute 58% of all drug offenders in state prisons (Drug Policy, 2002). The reasons for the disparity between drug use and incarceration are complex, but in large part they reflect two distinct approaches to the problem of substance abuse–a public health approach emphasizing treatment in middle-income communities and a law enforcement approach utilizing incarceration in inner city neighborhoods.

High rates of imprisonment in black communities impose a direct effect on family structure. One of every 14 black children today has a parent who is behind bars, and over the course of a year, or the duration of childhood, the figures are considerably higher. How does this affect the fourth grader who is "acting out" in class, trying to cope both with the absence of a parent and the stigma brought upon the family? How do these dynamics affect African Americans' attainment of social equality? How do they diminish faith in the fairness of law and the courts?

In the U.S., the direct effects of mass incarceration are increasingly being experienced by young people. Fear of "out-of-control" boys and girls and "super-predators" has undermined the traditional practice of treating young offenders as different from adults–less culpable and more amenable to rehabilitation because of their age. In recent years, the focus of juvenile policy has turned to punishment and in particular to the increasing transfer of youthful offenders from juvenile to criminal courts. As one report has argued, these "solutions" have shown to be doing more harm than good and to be doing nothing to increase public safety (Gainsborough & Young, 2000).

A recent study by Building Blocks for Youth shows that youth in Latino communities are increasingly singled out by the criminal justice system. The report details how harsh and disparate treatment at all stages of the justice system (including police stop, arrest, detention, waiver to adult criminal court, and sentencing) is a grim reality for many Latino youth who are part of the largest and fastest-growing racial/ethnic group in the United States. Furthermore, racial and ethnic disparities in the juvenile system are compounded by an unprecedented rate of construction of new juvenile facilities, jails and prisons across the country (Villaruel et al., 2002).

Perhaps one of the most dangerous effects of mass incarceration is the potentially explosive class division it is creating and sustaining. In a 1990 report titled *The Urban Underclass: Disturbing Problems Demanding Attention*, the U.S. General Accounting Office raised a red flag about class in America, putting forth the claim that a new underclass is firmly forming in U.S. society, in all geographic areas and concentrated in urban neighborhoods (US GAO, 1990). More recently, Robert Perrucci and Earl Wysong have demonstrated that the mid-twentieth century "middle-class" of U.S. society exists mostly as myth, and has actually been transformed into a bifurcated and polarized two-class society of a "privileged class" and a "new working class" (Perrucci & Wysong, 1999). In *The New Class Society* they argue that access to generative capital distinguishes the privileged class (20% of the population) from the new working class (80% of the population), whose environment has become increasingly unstable and unpredictable.

Paul Kingston takes issue with the notion that vast and persistent economic inequalities are evidence of social classes (Kingston, 2000). For this author modern occupational and technological developments have voided the foundations of class formation characteristic of early capitalism. Kingston presents abundant evidence showing the weakness or actual inability of class to predict labor market position, attitudes, politics, cultural tastes, or social networks. Nonetheless, such a position begs the more important question of inequality and its real life consequences. For example, in the recent Enron debacle, while some in management became millions of dollars richer, many workers lost their life savings or retirement funds. As Erik Olin Wright contends, it is simple-minded to argue that there are no real social classes with deeply opposing interests (Wright, 1997). His comparative study of sixteen industrial societies demonstrates the permeability of class boundaries and the ubiquity of class struggle and class-consciousness despite what is often the hegemonic triumph of one class over another.

But what is the connection between mass incarceration and social class? Simply that a whole section of the new working class exists in economic devastation, and constitutes the main feeder of the prisons and jails of this country. In fact, studies of class and the criminal justice system, such as Jonathan Simon's study of parole in the 20th century, show a direct relationship between class and imprisonment and argue that historically incarceration has been used to discipline the poor and those socially defined as "dangerous" (Simon, 1994). Simon and others are alarmed at the potential danger of such pointed class conflict, and warn of a future where we must choose "between a new reconstruction and a new civil war."

The economic effects on communities are profound as well. Ex-offenders returning to the community with a prison record find themselves competing for low-wage, low-skill employment. In broad terms, this translates into less economic and social capital in low-income communities, and thus the beginning of a vicious cycle that creates the underpinnings of neighborhoods where crime may flourish.

The morally questionable practice of prison privatization that profits from mass incarceration highlights the different meanings incarceration has come to have. Now a $2 billion industry, there were a reported 87,000 state and federal prisoners in private prison beds by 2000 (Greene, 2002). While three-strike offenders in California are given sentences of 25 years to life for theft of videotapes and golf clubs, on Wall Street millions are invested in private prisons in search of profit from such offenders. Private prison operators have approached state and federal governments with the promise of building and operating prisons at lowered costs, as well as providing the opportunity to avoid having to issue bonds for prison construction. But the advent of prison privatization raises a host of concerns regarding the fundamental fairness and appropriateness of contracting out the deprivation of liberty to an entity that is obligated to maximize return to its stockholders. Indeed, one recent newswire suggests "Investors looking for a safe place to lock-up an investment may want to consider the corrections industry" (McCarty, 2002).

The punitive approach to social policy represented by mass incarceration has expanded to related areas of policy, often in ways that are dramatically at odds with effective crime fighting approaches. One such step is the Federal Omnibus Crime Bill of 1994, which includes a provision that prohibits inmates from receiving Pell grants to pursue college education while in prison. Prior to the bill, the relative handful of prisoners with a high school degree and motivation to attend college could take advantage of college courses offered at prisons in many states by local institutions of higher education. Nationally, less than one percent of all Pell grant money went to support such programs. But in an act that can only be characterized as mean spirited, Congress cut this funding source.

In the absence of federal funding, prison college programs in many states have disappeared. Only one year after the Omnibus Crime Bill went into effect, more than half of the existing post-secondary correctional education (PSCE) programs reported very significant to completely changed programs, and three-quarters of existing programs reported a loss in student enrollment, with over a third measuring the loss in the hundreds (Tewksbury & Taylor, 1996). Student enrollment decreased 44%, and the 772 prisons that have PSCE programming have reported an enrollment shift from 38,000 inmate students to 21,000 inmate students (Tewksbury, Erickson, & Taylor, 2000).

Since research has consistently shown that education is associated with reduced recidivism, this policy can be called "anti-criminal" but certainly not "anti-crime." Adult educators have long argued that education provides critical reflection that leads to transformative learning, and as such serves both prisoners and society at large (Mezirow, 1990). However, given the continuing crunch felt by corrections budgets from expanding populations and the politically and popularly perceived "coddling" factors of prisoners receiving education, the future of PSCE programs looks bleak.

Congress has continued the excesses of the "war on drugs" as part of the passage of welfare reform legislation. A little-noticed provision of the 1996 bill stipulated that anyone convicted of a felony drug offense would henceforth be barred from receiving welfare benefits for life, unless individual states opted out of the provision. Thus, under the logic of this policy a three-time armed robber who is released from prison is eligible for welfare benefits but not a struggling single mother who engages in a one-time drug sale. As of December 2001, 22 states were enforcing the ban fully and 20 in part (Allard, 2002). Here, the impact of national policy is to make it even more difficult–for the largely female prisoners returning home after serving a drug sentence–to receive temporary welfare assistance to make the transition back to family life.

There is little likelihood that such a welfare ban policy will have any deterrent effect on drug selling, but it is quite certain that it will have deleterious effects on many poor women, children and communities, with a disparate impact on African American women and Latinas. Currently, over 92,000 women are affected by the lifetime welfare ban which places over 135,000 children at risk of coming in contact with child welfare services and the criminal justice system–due to the prospect of reduced family income (Allard, 2002).

The loss of welfare benefits adversely affects the ability of women, especially women of color, to become self-sufficient, provide for their children, and be active participants in their communities. The ban endangers the basic needs of low-income women and their children, including housing, food, job training, education and drug treatment, which are all key ingredients to help poor families lift themselves out of poverty. The ban is also likely to lead to higher incidences of family dissolution and further increases in child welfare caseloads, with enormous accompanying fiscal and social costs.

The movement toward mass incarceration is also affecting our democratic processes in ways that are increasingly profound. One such impact is through policies that strip away voting rights of convicted felons. Each state has its own policies in this regard, but in 48 states prisoners are not eligible to vote, in 32 states felons on probation and/or parole are excluded, and in 13 states ex-felons who have completed their sentence can still be barred from voting, in most cases for life (Felony Disenfranchisement, 2002). Thus, for example, an 18-year-old in Virginia who is convicted for selling drugs to an undercover agent is forever barred from the ballot box even if the youth lives a crime-free life. The only means of regaining voting rights is through a gubernatorial pardon, a time-consuming and cumbersome process in many states that frequently yields no results.

While these laws have existed in some states since the founding of the nation, the scale of imprisonment today results in disenfranchisement rates that are far from trivial. Nationally, about four million Americans–two percent of the voting age population–are currently barred from voting due to a current or prior felony conviction (Fellner & Mauer, 1998). Among African American males the rates are much higher, an estimated 1.4 million citizens, or 13% of that population (Fellner & Mauer, 1998). In the historic 2000 presidential election, the exclusion of at least 400,000 ex-felons in Florida was clearly of such magnitude as to have potentially altered the course of the election.

THE EMERGING PRACTICES OF RESTORATIVE JUSTICE

It is evident that current practices of mass incarceration are coming at a huge social cost. Many justice professionals, activists and academics are calling for proactive strategies that aim for prevention, or for redress of deep-seeded social problems. In many ways, this is a time ripe for the exploration of alternative strategies in response to crime and deviancy.

Much of the new thinking in this direction has come from the restorative justice movement. Restorative justice refers to a collection of practices that aim to address more than the punishment of the offender, and includes strategies such as community courts, reparation boards, community accountability conferencing, youth justice committees, mediation, community sentencing panels, releasing circles, healing lodges restorative justice dialogue, etc.

The advantage of the restorative justice paradigm is its three-dimensional view of crime and its focus on the needs of all parties: victims, community and offenders. In comparison, the traditional model acts only to punish offenders and in the process most often neglects the needs of both victims and the wider community, and the help they can provide. In the traditional paradigm, crime amounts to a violation of a state and its laws, offender accountability means punishment, and the system is designed on a winner/loser model. In the restorative justice paradigm, crime amounts to much more: Crime acts are also a violation of people and relationships, accountability also means offenders must understand the impact of their crimes and the need/opportunity to repair the harm. Finally, restorative justice functions on a model of participation of all parties and dialogue.

The inclusive nature of restorative justice addresses aspects of social justice that have not been appropriately incorporated yet in our justice system. It considers public safety beyond incarceration with accountability and competency development for offenders, searching for ways for them to make amends, repairs and ways to learn about the impact of their crime. It involves victims and makes them part of the decision-making and restoration process. Importantly, restorative justice brings the larger community to the table, involving the larger group in decision making, creating ownership, and making us all the caretakers of justice.

The growing restorative justice movement may represent a swinging of the pendulum away from the policy of mass incarceration that in the end has little to show in terms of citizen satisfaction or lowered recidivism. As such, restorative justice offers a template for an evolution of problem solving that goes beyond punishment. As law enforcement finds its resources strapped by increasing demands in new areas, as costs of corrections encroach on other funding needs, and as budgets are scaled back, victim and community involvement along with alternatives to incarceration can become key partners.

CONCLUSION

The scope of the effects of incarceration might be viewed by some as merely unfortunate by-products of an otherwise necessary approach to crime. But we have seen in recent years that there are far more effective, and socially less destructive, ways to affect crime. In Boston, a collaborative effort between criminal justice agencies and community groups has resulted in an impressive reduction in youth violence. In states across the country, drug courts are now diverting addicted offenders into court-supervised treatment rather than prison and jail terms. Many communities are engaged in restorative justice programs that bring together victims and offenders to engage in a process of fashioning appropriate ways for offenders to make victims whole again while also addressing the underlying factors contributing to crime.

As we have seen, crime is a complex social problem demanding careful and mindful consideration. We have also seen that solutions to crime require prudent study, as thoughtless responses to crime can and have worsened or transposed on to other social problems. We have seen that no single program or approach in itself offers a panacea to crime. Rather, what is becoming increasingly clear is that the American fixation on incarceration is having a broad set of consequences for the health of our society. To acknowledge this does not suggest that crime is not a legitimate concern for all Americans but rather to encourage a reassessment of how we address this problem in a way that draws on the strengths of families and communities rather than exacerbating their fragility.

The nation is engaged in ongoing efforts to combat the problems posed by HIV/AIDS and crime. The assumptions and values that we bring to these issues are critical in determining the public policy approaches that are employed. If we continue to perceive crime as essentially representing a failure of the criminal justice system, then the "answer" to the problem lies in the direction of tinkering or expanding the justice system. But if we view the problem instead as one that reflects a complex set of social and economic relationships, then we are obligated to envision a more comprehensive approach to its resolution. How we as a society respond to this choice will determine not only the relative use of imprisonment in the future, but also the health and vitality of our communities.

REFERENCES

Allard, P. (2002). *Life sentences: Denying welfare benefits to women convicted of drug offenses.* Washington, DC: The Sentencing Project.

Bonczar, T. & Beck, A. (1997). "Lifetime Likelihood of Going to State or Federal Prison." Washington: Bureau of Justice Statistics, U.S. Department of Justice.

Bureau of Justice Statistics (BJS) Bulletin. (May 1981). "Prisoners in 1980" (p. 2). Washington: U.S. Department of Justice.

Bureau of Justice Statistics (BJS) Bulletin. (1996). "Correctional Populations in the United States 1994" (pp. 10-13). Washington: U.S. Department of Justice.

Bureau of Justice Statistics (BJS) Bulletin. (2000a). "Prisoners in 1999" (pp. 10-12). Washington: U.S. Department of Justice.

Bureau of Justice Statistics (BJS) Bulletin. (2002). "Prison and Jail Inmates at Midyear 2001." Washington: U.S. Department of Justice.

Bureau of Justice Statistics (BJS) Bulletin. (1991). "Jail Inmates, 1990." (p. 4). Washington: U.S. Department of Justice.

Bureau of Justice Statistics (BJS) Bulletin. (2000b). "Prison and Jail Inmates at Midyear 1999" (p. 10). Washington: U.S. Department of Justice.

Caulkins, J. et al. (1997). "Mandatory Minimum Drug Sentences: Throwing Away the Key or the Taxpayer's Money?" (pp. xvii-xviii). Santa Monica, California: RAND Corporation.

Dickey, W. (1996). *The impact of "Three Strikes and You're Out" laws: What have we learned?* Washington, DC: Campaign for an Effective Crime Policy.

Dickey, W. & Hollenhorst, P. (1998). "Three Strikes five years later." Washington, DC: The Sentencing Project.

"Drug Policy and the Criminal Justice System." (2002). Washington, DC: The Sentencing Project.

"Facts About Prisons and Prisoners." (2002). Washington, DC: The Sentencing Project.

Fellner, J. & Mauer, M. (October 1998). "Losing the Vote: The Impact of Felony Disenfranchisement Laws in the United States." (p. 7). New York: Human Rights Watch and The Sentencing Project.

"Felony Disenfranchisement Laws in the United States." (April 2002) (p. 13). Washington, DC: The Sentencing Project.

Freeman, R. & Rodgers, W. (April 1999). "Area Economic Conditions and the Labor Market Outcomes of Young Men in the 1990's Expansion." Working Paper No. w7073. Cambridge, Massachusetts: National Bureau of Economic Research.

Gainsborough, J. & Mauer, M. (2000). "Diminishing Returns: Crime and Incarceration in the 1990s." Washington, DC: The Sentencing Project.

Gainsborough, J. & Young, M. (2000). "Prosecuting Juveniles in Adult Court, An Assessment of Trends and Consequences." Washington, DC: The Sentencing Project.

Greene, J. (2002). "Entrepreneurial Corrections: Incarceration as a Business Opportunity," in Mauer, M. & Chesney-Lind, M., eds., *Invisible punishment: The collateral consequences of mass imprisonment* (p. 95). New York: The New Press.

King, R. & Mauer, M. (2001). *Aging behind bars: "Three Strikes seven years later."* Washington, DC: The Sentencing Project.

Kingston, Paul. (2000). *The classless society.* Stanford, California: Stanford University Press.

Lynch, J. (1995). "Crime in an International Perspective," (pp. 11-38) in Wilson, J. & Petersilia, J., eds., *Crime.* San Francisco, CA: Institute for Contemporary Studies.

Mauer, M. (1999). *Race to incarcerate* (p. 9). New York: The New Press.

McCarty, P. (June 17, 2002). "Corrections Industry: Safe Place to Lock Away Investments." *Dow Jones Newswire.*

Mezirow, J. (1990). "How Critical Reflection Triggers Transformative Learning and Emancipating Education," in Mezirow, J. & Associates, eds., *Fostering critical reflection in adulthood.* San Francisco, CA: Jossey-Bass.

Perrucci, R. & Wysong, E. (1999). *The new class society.* Lanham: Rowman and Littlefield.

Rehnquist, W. (1993). June 18, 1993 Luncheon Address. In *Proceedings of the inaugural symposium on crime and punishment in the United States 286,* United States Sentencing Commission.

Rosenfeld, R. (2000). "Patterns in Adult Homicide," in Blumstein, A. & Wallman, J., eds., *The crime drop in America* (pp. 130-163). New York: Cambridge University Press.

Simon, J. (1994). *Poor discipline: Parole and the social control of the underclass, 1890-1990.* Chicago: University of Chicago Press.

Spelman, W. (2000). "The Limited Importance of Prison Expansion," in Blumstein, A. & Wallman, J., eds., *The crime drop in America* (pp. 97-129). New York: Cambridge University Press.

Tewksbury, R. & Taylor, J. (1996). "The Consequences of Eliminating Pell Grant Eligibility for Students in Post-Secondary Correctional Education Programs." (pp. 60-63) *Federal Probation,* v. 60 No. 3.

Tewksbury, R., Erickson, D., & Taylor, J. (2000). "Opportunities Lost: The Consequences of Eliminating Pell Grant Eligibility for Correctional Education Students." (pp. 43-56). *Journal of Offender Rehabilitation,* v. 31 (1/2).

U.S. General Accounting Office (US GAO). (1990). *The urban underclass: Disturbing problems demanding attention* (p. 1). GAO HRD 90-52, 1990.

United States Sentencing Commission (May 2002). *Report to Congress: Cocaine and Federal Sentencing Policy.*

Villaruel, F. et al. (2002). *¿DÓNDE ESTÁ LA JUSTICIA? A Call to Action on Behalf of Latino and Latina Youth in the U.S. Justice System*. Washington, DC: Building Blocks for Youth.

Vincent, B. & Hofer, P. (1994). *Mandatory minimum prison terms: A summary of recent findings*. Washington, DC: Federal Judicial Center.

Wright, E. (1997). *Class counts: Comparative studies in class analysis*. Cambridge: Cambridge University Press.

Families and the Moral Economy
of Incarceration

Donald Braman

SUMMARY. The experiences of families of prisoners barely register in contemporary debates over criminal sanctions. But the accounts of families of prisoners demonstrate that mass incarceration does far more than punish and deter. By pitting the moral and economic interests of families against one another, it erodes the fundamental norms of social life itself. As family members are pressed hard to withdraw their care and concern from one another, the effect is more than the impoverishment of individuals: As over-incarceration increases the costs of caring relationships, the loss becomes a moral one and, in time, we impoverish our culture as well. *[Article copies available for a fee from The Haworth Document Delivery Service: 1-800-HAWORTH. E-mail address: <docdelivery@haworthpress.com> Website: <http://www.HaworthPress.com> © 2004 by The Haworth Press, Inc. All rights reserved.]*

Donald Braman, PhD, is affiliated with Yale University (E-mail: donald.braman@ aya.yale.edu).

This research was funded by the National Institute of Justice (Award Number 98-CE-VX-0012), the National Science Foundation (Award Number SBR-9727685), the Wenner-Gren Foundation for Anthropological Research, and the Yale Center for the Study of Race, Inequality, and Politics. This research also could not have been conducted without the cooperation of the District of Columbia, Virginia, and Maryland Departments of Correction, and the various federal agencies working with District inmates.

[Haworth co-indexing entry note]: "Families and the Moral Economy of Incarceration." Braman, Donald. Co-published simultaneously in *Journal of Religion & Spirituality in Social Work* (The Haworth Social Work Practice Press, an imprint of The Haworth Press, Inc.) Vol. 23, No. 1/2, 2004, pp. 27-50; and: *Criminal Justice: Retribution vs. Restoration* (ed: Eleanor Hannon Judah, and Rev. Michael Bryant) The Haworth Social Work Practice Press, an imprint of The Haworth Press, Inc., 2004, pp. 27-50. Single or multiple copies of this article are available for a fee from The Haworth Document Delivery Service [1-800-HAWORTH, 9:00 a.m. - 5:00 p.m. (EST). E-mail address: docdelivery@haworthpress.com].

KEYWORDS. Children, families, incarceration, child development, criminal justice, policy

INTRODUCTION: HALFWAY THERE

Londa and her three children live in a small row house that is part of a Section Eight housing project in central Washington, DC. Inside her home, surrounded by the debris of family life–toys, a few empty kid-sized boxes of juice, dishes on the table from a lunch just finished, bottles and baby blankets strewn over the couch–she is apologetic for the mess. "But," she tells me, "I've got three kids, a broken leg, and a husband who's locked up." She has been struggling against her husband's crack addiction and struggling to keep her family together for fifteen years. Gesturing out the window, she says, "I don't want to end up like everyone else. I guess I'm halfway there. But my kids need a father. I look around here and none of these kids have fathers. It's a mess what's happened."

Londa's family is one of fifty families that participated in a study of incarceration and family life in the District of Columbia from 1998 to 2001 (Braman, 2002). Over the years that I have known her, Londa has repeatedly questioned her commitment to her husband, Derrick. She sees their current relationship as the culmination of her long struggle with his drug addiction and incarceration, a struggle that has left her feeling utterly drained and Derrick with years ahead of him in prison, both of them unsure of what kind of father he'll be able to be to his children.

While all families are unique, Londa and Derrick's story illustrates many of the themes that ran through the accounts of other families in this study, providing a fair account of the broad array of concerns that families of prisoners face. Derrick has been in and out of prison and addiction for over a decade. Like most of the inmates added to our criminal justice system in recent years, Derrick is a nonviolent offender (Mauer, 1999). Like most offenders who use drugs, he has neither been sentenced to nor received anything approaching serious treatment. As a result, like most prisoners, he is also a repeat offender (BJS, 2002). Perhaps most significantly, he, like most inmates, is also a father and, like most incarcerated fathers, both lived with his children prior to incarceration and remains in contact with them now (Mumola, 2000).

Derrick and Londa's story, neither one of flagrant injustice nor triumph against the odds, shows a family facing addiction, the criminal justice system's response to it, and the mixture of hardship and relief that incarceration brings to many families of drug offenders. Stories like theirs are almost entirely absent from current debates over incarceration rates and accountability. Indeed, the historical lack of the familial and community perspective of those most affected by incarceration can help to explain the willingness of states to accept mass-incarceration as a default response to social disorder. Once we begin attending to the accounts of people directly affected by criminal sanctions, however, we can begin to understand how our policies have exacerbated the very social problems they were intended to remedy. By not holding offenders accountable to their families and communities, incarceration–at least as it is currently practiced–frustrates the fundamental norms of reciprocity that form the basis of social order itself.

This article unfolds in four parts. Part I describes the extent of incarceration, its distribution in the District of Columbia, and some of the factors that have contributed to the historically high rates of crime and incarceration there and across the nation. Part II describes the difficulties that Derrick's family faced during his addiction and repeated incarcerations. Part III describes the material consequences that mass incarceration and lack of drug treatment has brought for families like Derrick's. Part IV describes how incarceration has altered the moral life of at-risk families, often creating material incentives that run counter to their moral concerns.

PART I: THE SETTING

Nearly every long-time resident of the District of Columbia can name friends or family members who have been or are presently incarcerated, and many have themselves spent time in jail or prison. Our nation's capital city, a place of residence and work for many national policy makers who draft the federal criminal codes and sentencing guidelines that directly affect poor urban communities, is also a prime example of the recent dramatic expansion of the criminal justice system nationwide.

The simple effects of these sentencing reforms, the ones we need only numbers to tell us about, begin to indicate the scope of the issue. In the District of Columbia, during the time of this study, about one out of every ten adult black men was in prison, and over half of the black men between the ages of 18 and 35 were under some type of correctional supervision (Lotke, 1997). About seven percent returned from prison over the course of each year, and most returned to the families and neighborhoods they lived in prior to their arrests. If these conditions persist, a substantial majority of the black men in the District and nearly all the men in the poorest neighborhoods can expect to be incarcerated at some time in their lives (Braman, 2002).

These are stunning statistics. Yet, the District is neither unusually harsh in its sentencing practices nor does it have a particularly high incarceration rate. Compared with other cities, incarceration in Washington is about average. Across the nation, over the last 20 years, arrests, convictions, and sentences have all risen, as tremendous resources have been devoted to expanding criminal codes, imposing longer sentences, hiring new officers and staff, and building new facilities to judge, classify and hold offenders (Donziger, 1995; Miller, 1996).

One of the most difficult questions criminologists have had to wrestle with is why the dramatic increase in the prison population has not been accompanied by a dramatic decrease in the crime rate. Despite the fact that our incarceration rate has more than tripled since 1960, the crime index remains at over twice what it was at that time.

Broadening the focus to include the effects of public policy on family life during this same period, however, can help make sense of the statistics. The 1960s, 70s, and 80s saw major federal cutbacks in programs and tax breaks benefiting parents—particularly married parents—with dependent children (Hewlett & West, 1988). And, at the same time, both liberals and conservatives supported the massive physical reordering of American cities and suburbs that shuffled poor families from bad homes to worse in cities like Washington. From redevelopment and highway construction to tax restructuring and housing incentives to the regulation of direct benefits, liberals and conservatives targeted one another, but hit poor families, particularly those in our inner cities.

As public policy exerted a steady corrosive force on family life in poor inner-city communities, crime rates (unsurprisingly) rose, fluctuating at about three to four times the rate measured in 1960 (see Figure 1).

The response to the historically high crime rate, both in the District and across the nation, has been a consistent increase in the use of incarceration as a sanction. In the District, as in jurisdictions across the nation, the movement towards longer and more rigidly determined sentences was achieved largely through a series of federal programs offering billions of dollars in federal aid during the last two decades:

1984 Comprehensive Crime Act & Sentencing Reform Act

Established mandatory minimum sentences for some federal drug offenders; abolished parole for all federal offenders; and required federal judges to use new sentencing guidelines.

1986 Anti-Drug Abuse Act

Established mandatory minimums for all federal drug offenders and transferred sentencing power from federal judges to prosecutors. Provided $1.7 billion to states for new prison construction.

1988 Omnibus Anti-Drug Abuse Act

Established mandatory minimums of five years for possession of five grams of crack cocaine and 20 years for continuing criminal enterprises, and broadly expanded conspiracy.

1994 Violent Crime Control and Law Enforcement Act (VOI/TIS)

Established 20 sentencing reforms, including mandatory sentencing and lengthened minimum sentences for drug offenses.

1996 Violent Offender Incarceration/Truth in Sentencing Act

Amending the 1994 Violent Crime Act, encouraged States to adopt federal sentencing guidelines with over 9 billion dollars in incentives for adopting new sentencing guidelines.

The District, ahead of many other jurisdictions, began to implement mandatory minimum sentencing in the early 1980s for violent offenders, then drug offenders, and, later, repeat offenders (Kiernan & Kamen, 1982). Most recently, in response to VOI/TIS funding opportunities, the District has also adopted both determinate and "truth in sentencing" measures (Tucker, 2000).

The ineffectiveness of sentencing reform in reducing criminal activity is particularly apparent in neighborhoods like Londa's. The area where Londa lives was devastated first by the 1968 riots, then by the heroin epidemic in the 1970s, declining public investment during the 1980s, and crack cocaine during the 1990s (Berry, 1997). Despite the efforts of numerous city and neighborhood organizations, the block she lives on is known today, as it has been for years, as a place where crack and heroin can be found on any street corner and at any hour (see Figure 2).

FIGURE 1. Crime in the US and Washington, DC

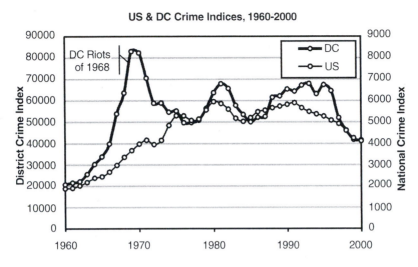

FBI (1960-2000)

During 1998, there were 64 arrests for drug possession and distribution within a two-block radius of her residence. Over 120 men living within the same two block radius were admitted to the DC Correctional system during that time, about one-quarter of them on drug possession or distribution charges. Many others, like Derrick, were incarcerated on other charges related to drug addiction.

Criminologists may debate the influence that the expansion of incarceration has had on crime rates–but from anthropological perspective at least, the debate seems poorly framed. What is of real concern is not the statistical representation of or relationship between criminality and punishment, but how crime and punishment are related to the nature of everyday social interactions in the families and communities that they most directly affect. To understand that we need more than statistics can provide, for only in the details of real lives can we find how crime and punishment operate and what they mean.

PART II: DERRICK AND LONDA

In many ways, Derrick and Londa had a lot going for them. From early on, Derrick made reliable money performing manual labor: laying carpet, working construction–any job that he could get to help them

FIGURE 2. Arrests and Incarceration in the District

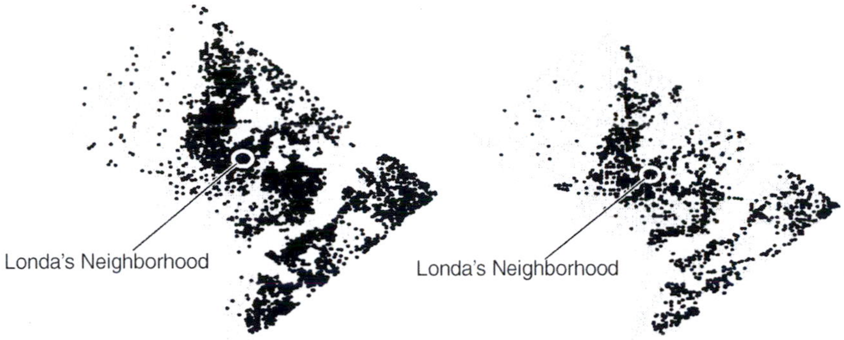

Residences of Male Prisoners (1998)   Drug Arrests (1998)

along. Unlike many young men in the neighborhood where he grew up, he knew that he could earn a living if he worked at it, and made it through his teens without any serious trouble. Londa, for her part, was a good student and, after high school, able to get work as a secretary. It wasn't long before Londa was pregnant. Derrick was 22 and Londa, 21.

Around the same time that Londa became pregnant, though, Derrick's drug use, once limited to the occasional party, became more serious. By the time their daughter was born in 1987, Londa could see changes in Derrick as he started covering for his growing addiction. Anyone who has experienced addiction in the family will know the litany of problems that Londa encountered: mood swings, lying, erratic behavior, late night disappearances, pleading for money, and eventually stealing.

As Londa realized how serious things had become, she tried to hold Derrick accountable as a parent, something she felt that she deserved and their daughter needed: "You get yourself together [and you can see her, but] I don't think she should get less from you and more from me . . . The best you can do is to come over here like that? No. I'm sorry, she deserves more than that." Shortly after she cut him off from seeing their daughter, Derrick was arrested and sentenced to eighteen months on a possession charge.

Although Derrick did not enter drug treatment while he was incarcerated, he managed to stay off of drugs and felt like he had recovered from his addiction. Londa was surprised to see that Derrick once again seemed like the person she'd fallen in love with: "The old Derrick was back," and he was insisting that he had reformed his ways, writing long letters of regret, talking about his religious reform in prison, and suggesting that they get married.

Derrick's family also pleaded with Londa to give Derrick another chance. Concerned about Derrick's morale, they were worried that his isolation from Londa and his daughter would push him back into his drug use. Londa offers:

> I think when I got married I was thinking, too, that I really, really wanted this person that I knew. Not necessarily he had to be the same as that person or act the same way. I didn't want that person where the demons had taken over. You know? I just wanted my Derrick back.

Many women described the way that their partner's immediate family would encourage them to remain faithful during incarceration, often emphasizing that this was the time when "they need you most." Many, including Londa, already felt that way themselves–particularly if they had children or considered themselves a family. As one woman said of her child's incarcerated father, "We're family. You don't . . . you can't just say 'bye-bye.' Either you're family or you're not and if you are then you do what's right."

When Derrick was released, Londa did marry him and Derrick did work hard to provide for his family. Indeed, many family members said that he worked harder after his release than he had prior to his arrest. As his sister Brenda told me:

> Derrick is a workaholic when he's not on drugs. And he told me why he does it: to keep his mind off drugs. He wants to stay busy, because that's what he needs when he's first out. And like he told me, he also . . . he's scared of society. He says, "It's scary out here," because he don't want to go back to jail.

Unfortunately, Derrick's recovery lasted a little less than a year. Then he was back on drugs and back in jail, a cycle that he would repeat several times. He would attend NA meetings for a while, work hard, pay the bills, and then one day he would run into some "friends" and it was all over–another binge and another set of broken promises. The difficulty faced by Londa was increased as, over the next five years, their daughter was joined by two sons.

Addiction and Incarceration

Most of the offenders in this study, like most of the prisoners added to our prisons over the last 20 years, were incarcerated on drug-related offenses. The families I spoke with described a cycle that drug offenders who don't receive treatment often repeated. The addicted family member would be incarcerated on some minor charge (usually possession or larceny), given a year or so in prison without drug treatment, and then released on parole. As was the case with Derrick and Londa, the parole board would contact the family to make sure that the offender has a place to live and a supportive environment. Families, knowing full well that their relative received little or no drug treatment, are then in a bind: If the family does not agree to take him in, he will simply spend more time in jail or prison without treatment. If they do agree, they do so knowing that he is likely to relapse and re-offend. Unsurprisingly, most families—urged on by the pleadings of the incarcerated family member, and ever hopeful that they will be able help him through recovery—agree to have him released to their care. Thus the cycle of good intentions and promises, followed by relapse, deeper addiction, and then reincarceration goes on.

Families in this study describe the cycle as ending in one of two ways. That which they feared most is death, and many drug offenders do die—victims of a drug overdose, an illness secondary to their addiction, or violence. Over the three years of this study, in fact, three of the fifty offenders that participated died drug-related deaths. But a fair number survive, and their cycle of abuse and incarceration ends another way: They commit a more serious offense or wear out the patience of a judge, garnering a lengthy sentence and, if not dying in prison, are released late in life (Robertson, 1997).

While it is too early to say for sure, the latter appears to be what is likely to happen in Derrick's case. After receiving several sentences for which he served less than two years apiece, Derrick found himself in front of an unsympathetic judge who simply saw no reason why this time would be any different. And so, what might have garnered a suspended sentence or parole for a first-time offense got him eight to twelve years.

There are, of course, far more desirable but also far less common ways of breaking the cycle. A very small proportion of offenders will be sentenced to mandatory drug treatment while incarcerated, followed by mandatory transitional treatment in a halfway house and then mandatory outpatient treatment. As a number of national studies have now demonstrated, this approach is highly effective when the quality of the treatment is high and the duration reasonably long (Gaes, Flanagan, Motiuk, & Stewart, 1999; The National Center on Addiction and Substance Abuse, 1998). And, despite the widely held belief that treatment must be voluntary to be successful, this same research has demonstrated that mandatory treatment is as successful as voluntary (Travis, 1999).

The issue is not a trivial one. Over 40% of the District's offenders test positive for illegal drugs, and over seventy percent report current or recent drug use (Drug Strategies, 1999). While mandatory treatment would thus seem to be an attractive sentencing option for judges and offenders alike, the chances of such a sentence being handed down and treatment being provided are slim. Even those judges who support treatment confront the practical reality that treatment–both in the correctional setting and in the community–is frustratingly scarce. As Faye Taxman, a University of Maryland professor who studies the District observed:

> [P]robably half of the sentences for probation have drug treatment required, but probably only ten percent get any type of services, and I use the word "services" lightly. The system has been structured to provide the minimum. We provide something less than the minimum and say we are providing services. (Slevin, 1998:A01)

Indeed, while it is estimated that 65,000 District residents need drug treatment, well over 80% cannot be placed because of lack of treatment facilities (Slevin, 1998).

The lack of available drug treatment also creates unintended incentives for inmates to avoid admitting to a drug problem and submitting to drug treatment as part of their sentencing. Because inmates can wait months–or even years–to gain entry into a drug treatment program that is a requirement of their release, many try to avoid sentencing that includes treatment even if they believe it would help them. They would rather just do "straight time" and be released than sit on a waiting list for a nonexistent slot in a drug program (Slevin, 1998). As one inmate told me, "Then, at least, you know. This other way, you maybe get out, you maybe don't. And then even if you do get out, you have to deal with all the nonsense with your parole officer." This, of course, increases the likelihood that they will be returned to their family and community without treatment and will relapse into drug use.

Small People and Big People

Derrick will likely spend at least another eight years in Maryland and DC facilities, and it could be as much as 20. While he is not happy to be separated from his family, he acknowledges that there are some benefits to his being incarcerated in Maryland where there are drug treatment and job training programs available. He told me that he saw his "incarceration as taking a burden off of his family, and it is hard not to agree his current incarceration is, on the whole, better for his family than when he was out and using drugs.

But Derrick's sister Brenda views his predicament with less equanimity than he does, and her lament was one I heard from many family members of drug offenders. The cycle of release, relapse, and reincarceration is one that she thinks could and should have been avoided:

> It's hard when people don't have the income or know how to find people that you can talk to, to know how to get into them [a drug treatment program], because a lot of people don't want to listen to smaller people like us. And you just kneel down, and you pray, and you just ask God to lead you in the right way, and just watch over us. Well, it's hard. And you're trying to survive for yourself. And my kids, my family take care of my income and everything with my household, and it's difficult. Then he has a wife and his kids, who are on the other side of town, and they're suffering, too, you know.

> [Wealthy people] got people, big people, helping them, pulling them out of situations. And when people, little people, get like that, that's a different story. For them, they get thrown away in jail and locked up, while people that's on in high places, they'll take them somewhere privately to a program, and then they get clean. Then they're around positive people and live in positive areas. But they don't do the same thing for people that's small people–they just throw them away in jail instead of them trying to say, "Well, I can make a deal here. If you spend such and such time in jail, and then you go from jail to a program out somewhere, until you feel like you got it mentally together, until you prove to me that I can

trust you to go from step one, to step two, to step three." You know? That's what I believe. That's what I see. I mean, why they don't see that?

Clearly the efforts of police, judges, correctional officers, wardens, departmental administrators, congressmen, and citizens–all of which have produced our current correctional system–are not conspiracies against poor families and communities. And yet, one can see why, from the perspective of families dealing with the criminal justice system, it seems like the product of a willfully ignorant if not malicious effort rather than a beneficent one.

The complicated truth is that, for many drug offenders, arrest and conviction does offer them a chance at sobriety and a chance to reestablish the family relationships that they damaged while they were free. But, as with all the times that Derrick went through the system, incarceration is a hardship for the family and, without treatment, is often followed by the further hardship of relapse and re-incarceration. As more and more offenders are incarcerated on drug-related charges, and as drug treatment falls ever further behind the need for it, the disparities in the criminal justice system become increasingly bound up with the disparities in drug treatment. In both cases, people get the best their money can buy, and for those without money, for "small people," that is often nothing at all.

PART III: MATERIAL CONSEQUENCES

The cycle of incarceration followed by relapse and re-incarceration can have a devastating effect on families. Perhaps the most obvious effects of current criminal practices are material. Reviewing Londa's income and expenses, it becomes clear that her financial problems are directly related to the loss of Derrick's income and the additional costs that accompany his incarceration. She lives on a fixed income of $463 a month from public assistance. After $100 for rent and another $300 for groceries (which works out to less than $3 of food per day, per person), there isn't enough to pay for electricity, the phone, and transportation. She is far from lazy, but with two children and one infant, she doesn't have the resources to care for them herself. "Oh, I can't stand to ask anybody to help me with anything. So I really hate asking my mother now, but I can't walk, I can't get around. So it's just really, really hard right now."

Londa's mother helps care for the children, buys groceries, and even pays Londa's rent when things are tight. But her assistance is limited to what she herself can afford, and that is not much. Already, Londa feels she has asked for far too much and far too often from her mother. "I know that she doesn't have a lot, too, so that's something I have to think about." Derrick's sisters also try to help when they can, but they have families of their own and are struggling just to get by. Derrick's sister, Brenda, describes her surprise at how "it just all adds up." "The phone bills–the phone bill is something else!" One of the more unpleasant surprises to many families is the high cost of phone calls from prison. Inmates can only call collect, and additional charges for monitoring and recording by the prison phone company add up quickly; indeed, many families have their phones disconnected within two months of an incarceration.

Indeed, the most costly regular expense that families in this study complained about were phone charges. Most correctional facilities contract out phone services and actually receive money from the phone company for doing so. Phone companies thus compete with each other for the service, but not by providing lower prices: The key criteria that phone companies compete on is how much revenue the service will return to the Department of Corrections in each state. Because phone conversations are often time-limited, many families are required to accept several calls to complete a single conversation, with connection charges applying to each call. While there are no data on overall phone costs for DC inmates, the costs are high locally and nationally. As one news account has noted:

> In Florida, where the state prison system collected $13.8 million in commissions in fiscal 1997-98, a legislative committee found that big prison systems in ten other states took in more than $115 million in the same budget year. New York topped the list with $20.5 million. In Virginia, MCI gave the state $10.4 million, or 39 percent of the revenue from prison calls. Maryland receives a 20 percent commission on local calls by inmates, which must be made through Bell Atlantic, and gets 42 percent of revenue from long-distance calls, all of which are handled by AT&T. (Duggan, 2000)

As a result, collect calls from prisons can be as much as 20 times as expensive as standard collect calls.

Rather than risk another disconnect and a subsequent hefty reconnect fee, many families block calls from the prison because they cannot bring themselves to say no to the collect call. Families with loved ones incarcerated out of state have shown me years of phone records that average well over $200 a month. Many families in this study, including Londa's, have had their phone or electricity cut off for lack of payment.

After having her phone cut off for high bills the last time Derrick was incarcerated, Londa realized she had trouble refusing calls she couldn't afford and had a "block" placed on her phone preventing collect calls. In an arrangement that is not unusual, Derrick's sisters now serve as a conduit to his extended family; because no one else will accept the expense of collect calls from prison, they try to patch him through to whomever he needs to talk to using three-way calling. While it further increases the overall price of the call, it is another way for Derrick's family to spread the cost of his incarceration.

While Londa is fortunate to have family that are willing to help her in Derrick's absence, her family doesn't have much to help her with. By spreading the costs of raising Derrick's children and maintaining ties with him, Londa and Derrick's families have enabled Londa to keep and care for her children. While this is undoubtedly desirable, the cost has simply been spread to other low-income households with few resources, lessening the impact on any one person, but creating a steady drain on the extended family.

Londa, for example, can no longer afford her own car–an issue that became quite serious when her mother's car broke down and, largely as a result of helping Londa, her mother was unable to afford the repair costs. Derrick's sister, Brenda, has also struggled with the sacrifices that she makes to keep her brother in touch with his family.

> I'm gonna be there regardless of what. And his wife, well she's she having it rough, her and her kids, because, she don't have anything, which I don't have anything either, but a lot of times I [still help out]. My kids don't like it, because I try to give to [Derrick's family], because, you know . . . I . . . I feel for them and for him in that jail. [And] when school comes it's like, do my kids, do they get new shoes or does he get to talk to his kids. And, you know, I just think he needs to talk to them.

Families can be tremendous resources, but they are not limitless funds of wealth and generosity. The costs of Derrick's repeated incarcerations have been dear in both material and emotional terms.

Indeed, despite the emphasis on accountability when policy makers talk about the criminal justice system, Londa's story shows us how, in an attempt to punish criminality, policy makers have effectively held offenders like Derrick almost entirely *not* accountable in ways that matter a great deal. His enforced withdrawal from the economic responsibilities of family life has pushed both his and Londa's extended family more deeply into poverty. Given that they started with little, that loss has been all the more keenly felt.

More subtle than the immediate and direct material effects of incarceration on these families, but perhaps more serious, is the cumulative impact they can have on familial wealth across generations. By depleting the savings of offenders' families, incarceration inhibits capital accumulation and reduces the ability of parents to pass wealth on to their children and grandchildren through inheritance and gifts. Indeed, incarcerations draining of the resources of extended family members in this study–particularly the older family members–helps explain why there has been so little capital accumulation and inheritance among inner-city families in general and minority families in particular.

This becomes apparent when we see Derrick's family struggling to save enough to buy their children school supplies, let alone provide for their inheritance. The disproportionate incarceration of men such as Derrick helps to explain why black families are less able to save money and why each successive generation inherits less wealth than their white counterparts. Criminal sanctions–at least in their current form–act like a hidden tax, one that is visited disproportionately on poor and minority families, and while its costs are most directly felt by the adults closest to the incarcerated family member, the full effect is eventually felt by the next generation as well.

Viewed in this light, the racial disparities in arrests, sentencing, and parole described by Donziger (1996), Kennedy (1997), Currie (1988), Cole (2000), Mauer (1999), and Tonry (2001) take on a broader significance. For example, census data show that blacks typically possess only one-third the assets of whites with similar incomes (Lynch, 1988; Blau & Graham, 1990; Oliver & Shapiro, 1995). While this pattern is generally attributed to lower savings and inheritance (Smith, 1995; Avery & Rendall, 1997; Menchik & Jianakoplos, 1997), this explanation begs the question of why savings and inheritance are lower–something that the concentration of incarceration in minority communities and its effect on capital accumulation help to explain.[1] Finally, it is worth noting that familial costs can also decrease investments in what is often called "human capital" (Becker, 1981; England & Folbre, 1997), as moving to a better school district, purchasing an up-to-date computer, and attending college all become less affordable. Educational attainment is one of the best predictors we have for avoiding the criminal justice system; but the benefits of investing in (and the costs of neglecting) human capital extend well beyond crime rates. As the stock of resources that a family possesses diminishes, and as members are prevented from caring for one another, more than money and objects are lost. Indeed, the material losses these families face may, in the end, be the least significant concern.

PART IV: PULLING FAMILIES APART

In addition to material concerns are those respecting the integrity of the family itself, and it is here that incarceration's impact is perhaps most troubling. The difficulties involved in trying to visit Derrick, the expense of his calls, the wear and tear of untreated addiction are all things that Londa feels are pulling her and Derrick apart. In this way, the enforced imbalance of their relationship is coloring her perception of him and what he is capable of. While she still loves him dearly, Londa feels like fifteen years of struggling to hold her family together has taken its toll on her emotionally: Even though he may get treatment this time around, she is unsure of whether she can hold out hope for another eight years.

If Londa's patience is wearing thin, that of her own extended family is worn out. In this sense, it is not simply self-reliance that makes Londa reluctant to ask for help from her family: "My mother can't even hear me talk about him. She'll be like 'What? Are you crazy?'" His aunt tells Londa point blank that "He needs to stay where he is."

> She's just really, really bitter about it. And, I didn't know this until I spoke with her awhile back. And, I didn't know she felt like that. But she was really, really headstrong about him. "He needs to stay where he is and he better never come see me again." It's hard. Like he tells me a lot, he tries to make amends with people, and, he can't . . . And it's because, most people don't understand addicts. They just know that they are addicts and they don't want to have nothing to do with them.

Londa has largely stopped talking to her extended family about Derrick and tries not to ask for help except from Derrick's sisters–a point that begins to indicate how the economic impacts of incarceration are often bound up with its effects on family dynamics. For Londa, the material, emotional, and moral concerns are related in ways that she feels are straining her ties with both her own and her husband's families.

Londa's concerns also often turn to her three children–Sharon who just turned eleven, Cooper who is two, and DJ who is one. As hard as the cycle of addiction and incarceration has been for Londa, she feels it has been far harder for her daughter, who still has trouble understanding why her father could be loving and responsible one month but manipulative and reckless the next. "Trying to explain to a kid why her father left with her radio and why he's not allowed in the house at the moment, that's just not something a kid can really understand." The fact that Derrick, when sober, was a good father made the times that he wasn't all the harder. Londa described their relationship as a close one that has slowly deteriorated. But Londa doesn't think that her daughter ever forgot what it was like when Derrick was sober. "She really misses that, because when she was little they were really, really close."

In addition to missing her father and coping with her own ambivalence towards him, though, Sharon has also had to manage the information about her father in her encounters with friends and teachers. Londa believes that Derrick's incarceration has led her daughter, already a quiet girl, to become increasingly private and withdrawn.

> It bothers her because, you know, everybody is dealing with their fathers and school and their mothers. They come see them in show and stuff. [. . .] You could see the hurt. I mean it's not more or less she's gonna come out say it. She's gonna keep everything in 'til she can decide, "Okay, who do I want to talk to?" You know. Other than that, she really is very private. But I could see it. She has girlfriends and stuff, but they don't know.

> He told me that he was sending her a watch or something, and I didn't tell her. And when it came in the mail, I said "You got a package in the mail." But I wasn't really thinking about it. [. . .] She said "Oh it's from my father." I said "Um-hmm." And she opened it up. She said, "Oh look what he got me!" She was really, really happy about it. Then her friends came along and they were saying, "What's that?" "This is my new watch," and [her friend] said, "Oh that's cute. Where'd you get that?" She said, "My father gave it to me." [Her friend] said, "Your father gave it to you?

When?" And she said, "Yeah. What you think, I don't have no father?" No father. You know?

And then her schoolwork. It showed in her schoolwork. And my
daughter is a brain. You know. "A's" ever since she made kinder-
garten. She's never gotten a "C." Never. Fifth grade everything
just went [downhill]. He went to jail and everything just . . . she
just really went down this . . . And I know that in the fifth grade
year and I receive her report card and they said she had to repeat a
grade, I cried, I . . . I hurt. It bothers me now. It still bothers me.
You just think, you know, there is nothing that you can do. What
can you do?

While Derrick's sons are still quite young, his incarceration also
raises troubling questions about their development. Indeed, one of the
best predictors of male involvement in the criminal justice system is, of
course, the incarceration of a parent.

Londa looks back on the times that she had nothing and wasn't sure
how she would feed her kids, often sending them to stay with relatives
while she went to look for work. She feels like she has been torn between wanting to be a supportive wife and being a good mother to her
children, often feeling like she failed at the latter.

I feel like I let my kids down. I feel like I really *really* let them
down. And [this last time] I was out of work. I didn't have no
money. I felt like I was just getting exactly what I deserved and,
you know. Even all the good I did, it didn't outweigh the bad or
something. I just felt like I was just getting everything that I was
supposed to get. I was bitter. I didn't want to talk to nobody.

Londa's experience of depression and isolation was one that many
women I spoke with described as they tried to find some way to be a
good mother and a good partner without resources adequate to do either.

The last time I interviewed Derrick in person, he knew he was losing
Londa. He was struggling to figure out how to cut his time down or be
relocated near DC so that he could avoid losing touch with his family altogether.

My problem now is this. I got to choose between the treatment
route, the education route, and the job route. Now on the treatment
route, I'll get nothing [in the way of money]. Doing school, maybe

just enough to cover cosmetics, but that's it. I go the job route, and I can send home some money and, see, that helps out Londa and keeps the family intact. The point is, though, that they ain't coming to see me here and ain't taking my calls 'cause they can't afford the collect. But if I take the job, I don't get the drug treatment. So I'm trying to focus on the family, but I'm also kinda trying to get out of here. But it's also, too, I want to get back with them.

See, now I have two boys. One of them knows me but the other one was born while I was in here, and when I got out I only picked him up one time when he was a baby. And he's named after me, you know, but he don't know me, from Adam. His mother may show him some pictures and things and say, "This is your father," or whatever. Maybe, I don't know. But I think my oldest son, he do know me a little bit. He's four years old now, so he may not know me as well, or maybe my face or something, you know, remember it. Well, now since I'm in here, I try to be a father to them, sending them money, you know, to be able to help the mother out. [. . .] I try to do that, you know. So if I keep up the job, I can send back money, keep Londa a little more happy, keep the kids knowing me. But then I just go in circles. The judge said I have to do the treatment here before I go for parole. [. . .] I mean, I look at it and it would have been so easy to be a father out there. Maybe not easy, but it's like it's impossible here.

These issues weigh heavily on Londa, as she considers how much her commitment to Derrick has cost her. Perhaps the greatest loss that Londa has suffered is not material at all; it is the loss of her faith in the family itself. Looking back on her relationship with Derrick, she describes what many young women in her situation dream of:

I always thought that, "Okay, we want to raise our kids together." There's not too many [families], there's not any that I can think of at this time that's not a single-parent family. I never wanted that for my kids. I wanted them to have something that I didn't have. So you try to give them this and you try to give them that. But to me it is more important to have both your parents there. And I've always thought, you know, "Okay, that will happen." I always thought that would happen.

What is striking in Londa's and other accounts is the degree to which that dream, against all odds, remains alive–even if only as a dream. While she still holds out some faint hope that Derrick might be released early to a treatment program, she is exhausted from years of trying to work it out with Derrick. After this last incarceration, Londa reluctantly began considering filing for divorce.

> I mean, at first when we was dating, I could just walk away. But now, you know, I put a ring on my finger, and I'm married, and so it's more difficult now because I'm married to him. And I have more kids. I already had one, but I have more kids now. It would be a lot less pressure on me to stay, by me not being married to him.

None of the women and few of the men I met expressed a negative attitude towards marriage; most had marital ambitions but low expectations of achieving them–a finding consistent with a number of previous studies (Tucker, 2000; Manning & Smock, 1995; Brien & Lillard, 1999). While there are many factors involved in the increase of divorce and out-of-wedlock births over the last thirty years, the people I interviewed generally described marriage as not only a desirable goal, but also a serious commitment. Indeed, many wives of prisoners like Londa said that they would have left their partners had they not been married to them–a finding in keeping with the only longitudinal statistical study to date of incarceration's effect on family formation using individual-level data (Western & McLanahan, 2000).

Marital contracts and spousal exchanges are far more than casual agreements between consenting adults, freely entered or abandoned. Establishing and sustaining long-tem trusting relationships–relationships where the balance sheets are never fully closed or disclosed–helps people to get through hard times financially and emotionally and gives moral meaning to their lives. But these same relationships can exert a strong normative pull on those who are in them, spreading the harsh realities of addiction and incarceration far beyond criminal offenders.

Men in facilities where there is no employment are essentially dependent on their families to help them, but the bonds of family can only be stretched so far. By making marriage more difficult, incarceration lowers the likelihood that men and women will view marriage as a tenable or even desirable option. This effect is especially strong in pre-marital relationships, even where children are present; but as Londa's case illustrates, the meaning of marriage can change for those who have taken their vows as well.

The meaning of family to Londa remains powerful; but, given her long struggle with Derrick's addiction and her desire to achieve the middle-class status for herself and her children, that meaning came with a heavy price. Before asking whether, in hindsight, she was wise to bear the costs of that commitment, we might ask what the costs (both public and private) would be were she and others in poor inner-city families to decide that their commitments are too heavy to bear and withdraw their support, concern, and care from one another.

During incarceration, many prisoners and family members alike regularly question the concern that others had for them. By undermining not only the material ability of prisoners to reciprocate, but the sense of caring that inhabits reciprocal relationships, incarceration can increase the perception that individuals really do need to look out for themselves first, that others are inherently selfish, and that all relationships are inherently exploitative. While many wrestled with these perceptions and were able to maintain a trusting and caring relationship, others were not. The broader impact of that diminished trust is difficult to measure, but it may well outweigh all the material costs combined.

CONCLUSION: RETHINKING ACCOUNTABILITY

People like Londa don't often appear in accounts of the criminal justice system, but they have much to teach us. Their accounts begin to indicate how much many family members are willing to sacrifice in order to adhere to the norms that kinship engenders. It is, in a way, heartening that many family members are willing to bear high costs in order to show their dedication to one another. But families are not limitless trusts of generosity, and if the costs become great enough, the meaning of family itself can change or be lost.

In policy discussions, family and community life in our inner cities are described more often as a contradiction in terms rather than a realistic policy goal. Indeed, many commentators reason that if substantial family and community ties existed in our inner cities, our inner cities wouldn't have the kind of social problems that are now endemic there (Putnam, 1995; Fukuyama, 1999).

Unfortunately, the pervasive stereotype of an urban "underclass"–one that is uninterested in and unable to forge a coherent family or community life–has had significant practical effects. Policy makers, seeing no families or communities to protect in crime-stricken areas, have come to view residents of minority, urban, and low-income neighborhoods as somehow outside of and untouched by the social norms of society at large. The result has been a set of policies that, out of ignorance, have essentially given up on family and community life in the ghetto, attempting to maintain public order by using punitive sanctions in their stead.

Criminal policies are often justified with assertions of moral accountability. If the law is the embodiment of our collective will and sanctions the enforcement of our collective norms, then it is important to think carefully about how and to whom we are holding offenders accountable. Incarceration, the preferred punishment in American criminal law, does more than punish and deter. As the stories of prisoners' families make clear, incarceration also transforms the material and moral lives of many of the families it touches, often enforcing a lack of accountability in ways that are both meaningful and destructive. The current practice of mass incarceration thus does far more than inflict an overly harsh punishment. By prohibiting so many from engaging in basic moral behavior, it is cutting away at the basic building blocks of social life itself. As over-incarceration increases the costs of caring relationships, the loss becomes a social and a moral one. When individuals are pressed to withdraw their care and concern from one another, the effect is more than the impoverishment of individuals: In time, it is our culture itself that becomes impoverished.

NOTE

1. Incarceration, of course, is not alone in contributing to these disparities. Perhaps most obviously, the structure of our current welfare policies discourages capital accumulation by punishing savings with the discontinuation of assistance. This point was made forcefully by Carol Stack (1975) in her still resonant analysis of families living in a Chicago housing project. "Welfare policy effectively prevents the poor from inheriting even a pitifully small amount of cash, or from acquiring capital investment typical for the middle class, such as home ownership" (p. 127).

REFERENCES

Avery, R. B. & Rendall, M. S. (1997). *The Contribution of Inheritances to Black-White Wealth Disparities in the United States*. BLCC Working Paper #97-08.
Becker, G. S. (1981). *A Treatise on the Family*. Cambridge, MA, and London, England: Harvard University Press.

Berry, J. M. (1997). *BLS to Test Experimental CPI. The Washington Post,* April 11, 1997, p. G03.

BJS (Bureau of Justice Statistics) (2002). *Special Report, Recidivism of Prisoners Released in 1994.*

Blau, F. D. & Graham, J. W. (1990). *Black-White Differences in Wealth and Asset Composition. Quarterly Journal Of Economics,* 105:321-339.

Braman, D. (2002). *Families and Incarceration.* In M. Mauer & M. Chesney-Lind (Eds.), *Invisible Punishment,* 117-135.

Brien, M. J. & Lillard, L. A. (1999). *Interrelated Family-Building Behaviors: Cohabitation, Marriage and Non-Marital Conception. Demography,* 36:535.

Cole, D. (2000). *No Equal Justice.* New York: The New Press.

Currie, E. (1988). *Crime and Punishment in America.* New York: Henry Holt & Company.

DC DOC (1980-1996). *Population Reports.*

Donziger, S. (1996). *The Real War on Crime: The Report of the National Criminal Justice Commission.* New York, NY: HarperCollins Publishers, Inc.

Drug Strategies (1999). *Facing Facts: Drugs and the Future of Washington, DC.*

Duggan, P. (2000). *Captive Audience Rates High; Families Must Pay Dearly When Inmates Call Collect. Washington Post,* January 23, 2000, p. A03.

England, P. & Folbre, F. (1997). *Reconceptualizing Human Capital.* Paper presented at the annual meetings of the American Sociological Association, Toronto, Canada, August.

FBI (1960-2000). *Uniform Crime Reports.*

Fukuyama, F. (1999). *The Great Disruption.* London: Profile Books, Ltd.

Gaes, G. G., Flanagan, T. J., Motiuk, L. L., & Stewart, L. (1999). *Adult Correctional Treatment in Prisons. Criminal Justice: A Review of Research,* 25:361.

Gillette, Howard, Jr. (1995). *Between Justice and Beauty.* Baltimore: The Johns Hopkins University Press.

Kennedy, R. (1997). *Race, Crime, and the Law.* New York: Vantage Books.

Kiernan, Laura, A. & Kamen, Al (1982). *Crimes Involving Guns, Drug Sales; Mandatory Sentence Proposal Strongly Backed in D.C. Vote. The Washington Post,* September 15, 1982, A15.

Lotke, E. (1997). *Hobbling a Generation: Young African American Men in D.C.'s Criminal Justice System Five Years Later.*

Lynch, M. (1988). *Piece of the Pie. Reason Magazine,* July 1998.

Manning, W. D. & Smock, P. J. (1995). *Why Marry? Race Relations and Transition to Marriage Among Cohabitors. Demography,* 95:509.

Mauer, M. (1999). *Race to Incarcerate.* New York: The New Press.

Menchik, P. L. & Jianakoplos, N. (1997). *Black-White Wealth Inequality: Is Inheritance the Reason? Economic Inquiry,* 35:428-442.

Miller, J. G. (1996). *Search and Destroy: African-American Males and the Criminal Justice System.* New York: Cambridge University Press.

Mumola, C. J. (2000). *Bureau of Justice Statistics, Special Report, Incarcerated Parents and Their Children.*

Oliver, M. & Shapiro, T. (1995). *Black Wealth/White Wealth.* New York: Routledge.

Putnam, R. D. (1995). *Bowling Alone, America's Declining Social Capital. Journal of Democracy,* 6:1, p. 65-78.

Roberston, T. (1997). *How to Pay for Elderly Prisoners? Minneapolis Star Tribune,* January 20, 1997, p. 1B.

Slevin, P. (1998). In D.C., *Many Addicts and Few Services; Lack of Treatment Programs Keeps Substance Abusers in Jail or in Trouble. The Washington Post,* August 25, 1998, p. A01.

Smith, J. P. (1995). Racial and Ethnic Differences in Wealth in the Health and Retirement Study. *Journal of Human Resources,* 30:S158-83.

Stack, C. (1975). *All Our Kin.* New York: Harper Torchbooks.

The National Center on Addiction and Substance Abuse (1988). *Behind Bars: Substance Abuse and America's Prison Population.*

Tonry, M. (2001). *Malign Neglect.* New York: Oxford University Press.

Travis, J. (1999). *Addressing Drug Abuse in the Justice Context: The Promise and the Challenge, Remarks Before the National Assembly on Drugs, Alcohol Abuse, and the Criminal Offender.*

Tucker, M. B. (2000). *Marital Values and Expectations in Context: Results from a 21-City Survey.* In Linda J. Waite (Ed.), *The Ties That Bind.* New York: Aldine de Gruyter.

Western, B. & McLanahan, S. (2000). *Fathers Behind Bars: The Impact of Incarceration on Family Formation.* In G. L. Fox & M. L. Benson (Eds.), *Families, Crime and Criminal Justice.* New York: JAI/Elsevier.

Drug Policy:
A Challenge of Values

Eric E. Sterling

SUMMARY. This paper argues that the war on drugs is based on retributive values that are illogical, burden the criminal justice system, and are ineffective in reducing drug-related harm. It examines the relation between political agendas and anti-drug legislation. It demonstrates that anti-drug policy has resulted in dramatically inceased punishment and incarceration since 1970, after four decades at a level rate, especially for blacks. This paper contends that segregation was a form of nonjudicial punishment for blacks until 1970, and concludes tht the war on drugs has become a punishment substitute for segregation. It argues that drug prohibition must be replaced by regulation and that devising such a system involves a complex balance of competing values. *[Article copies available for a fee from The Haworth Document Delivery Service: 1-800-HAWORTH. E-mail address: <docdelivery@haworthpress.com> Website: <http://www.HaworthPress.com> © 2004 by The Haworth Press, Inc. All rights reserved.]*

KEYWORD. Drug policy, politics, punishment, race discrimination, restorative justice, segregation, war on drugs

Eric E. Sterling, JD, is President, Criminal Justice Policy Foundation, 8730 Georgia Avenue, Suite 400, Silver Spring, MD 20910-3649 (E-mail: esterling@cjpf.org).

The author gratefully acknowledges the assistance of Sanho Tree of the Institute of Policy Studies, and Anirudh Suri, Haverford College, '06, for locating and obtaining newspaper archives.

[Haworth co-indexing entry note]: "Drug Policy: A Challenge of Values." Sterling, Eric E. Co-published simultaneously in *Journal of Religion & Spirituality in Social Work* (The Haworth Social Work Practice Press, an imprint of The Haworth Press, Inc.) Vol. 23, No. 1/2, 2004, pp. 51-81; and: *Criminal Justice: Retribution vs. Restoration* (ed: Eleanor Hannon Judah, and Rev. Michael Bryant) The Haworth Social Work Practice Press, an imprint of The Haworth Press, Inc., 2004, pp. 51-81. Single or multiple copies of this article are available for a fee from The Haworth Document Delivery Service [1-800-HAWORTH, 9:00 a.m. - 5:00 p.m. (EST). E-mail address: docdelivery@haworthpress.com].

Humanitarianism consists in never sacrificing a human being to a purpose.

–Albert Schweitzer (1875-1965), 1923
Laureate
Nobel Peace Prize, 1952

In 1973, Blumstein and Cohen proposed a theory of the stability of punishment. They analyzed Durkheim's thesis that crime is a "normal" attribute of healthy societies and helps to maintain social solidarity because it contributes to the "collective conscience" or "the totality of beliefs and sentiments common to average citizens of the same society." Some read Durkheim and Kai Erickson to suggest that the level of crime "will rarely fall short of or exceed the relevant optimum." Blumstein and Cohen reexamined this premise to suggest that it is not crime so much as deviance that is punished, and that it is a constancy of punishment of deviance that exists. A key element of their hypothesis is that "if behavior were to become less deviant . . . then society would respond . . . by redefining previously minor infractions as crimes, and punishing these."

This paper argues that since the seventeenth century, to be black was to be deviant in the American "collective conscience" (Higginbotham, 1996; Kennedy, 1997, pp. 29-167), and that status has been punished through slavery, through segregation, and now through the criminal justice system, especially by means of the "war on drugs."

This thesis is important for understanding the consequences of involvement of drug control in the criminal justice system, and for understanding the relevance of drug policy reform to the reforms of restorative justice.

This paper weaves two twentieth-century phenomena. "The problem of the twentieth century is the problem of the color line," said W. E. B. DuBois famously, as Judge Higginbotham notes (1996, p. xxiv), and drug prohibition.

DRUG POLICY AND THE CRIMINAL JUSTICE SYSTEM

The idea of drug use and drug trafficking has generated fear throughout American society for more than a century (Musto, 1999). A statement attributed to Timothy Leary may be apocryphal but makes the point: "LSD (or marijuana, in some versions) is such a powerful drug, it has generated paranoia in persons who have never used it."

In fact, drug use and drug trafficking generate many problems (Kleiman, 1992; Ray & Ksir, 1999; Goode, 1999). MacCoun and Reuter (2001) have compiled a forty-eight-item taxonomy of drug-related harms, including seventeen criminal justice harms such as increased costs, corruption of legal authorities, court congestion and delay, stigma of criminal or prison record, etc. Other harms include overdoses by users, crimes by users to get money to buy drugs, violence and corruption by the traffickers, money laundering, dysfunction in the workplace and schools by users, etc. They note that harms are distributed to users, their intimates, their employers, to neighborhoods and to society at large, as well as to dealers (pp. 106-108).

Manski, Pepper and Petrie (2001) succinctly set forth the American approach to drug control:

> As traditionally conceptualized, the two prongs of drug control policy are supply reduction and demand reduction. Supply reduction is usually understood to be synonymous with enforcement of drug law prohibitions and international interdiction activities, whereas demand reduction is usually thought to encompass clinical treatment of drug abuse and addiction as well as the spectrum of activities aiming to prevent youths from using drugs (e.g., media campaigns, school-based education programs). This conceptualization is imperfect for two reasons. First, a large component of drug law enforcement focuses directly on reducing demand (e.g., apprehending and punishing users for possessing drugs). Second, the standard menu of demand-reduction activities tends to overlook (or take as given) the rich fabric of deeply ingrained social controls against illicit drug use, including legal controls. (p. 187)

Moore (2001, pp. 38-39) distinguishes four types of prevention: (1) social policies to change the environmental conditions fostering drug use (i.e., reducing poverty and racial discrimination, increasing employment, improving care of children); (2) changing the milieu of experimental users (i.e., providing after school activities, changing the views about drug use by teen subcultures); (3) supply reduction efforts to make it harder, more expensive and more dangerous to access drugs; and (4) policies to reduce the harm associated with a given level of drug use.

But Moore (2001, p. 19) argues that preventive effects of drug enforcement may be more effective and important in reducing drug use than the usually understood prevention programs.

Indeed, American society has overwhelmingly relied upon enforcement through the criminal justice system to prevent the problems caused by, associated with, and imagined to be caused by drug use as measured by dollar expenditures, personnel commitments, and persons affected (White House, 2002a, 2002b). Our approach has been ineffective in reducing drug use, saving lives, reducing crime, or hindering drug traffickers. One must ask what other purposes this failed policy serves. This paper argues that the policy not only serves the careers of politicians, but also carries forward the advantages of white privilege that existed in law before 1970 by invidiously punishing people of color (Lusane, 1991, pp. 25-53).

RETRIBUTION AGAINST USERS

Use of the criminal justice system to stop drug users is even more of a retribution-based system than the usual model. The typical sense of retribution in criminal justice is that punishment is inflicted against the perpetrator for an act that hurts an innocent person. In the "just desserts model," if you hurt someone, you deserve to be hurt in turn. In the deterrence model, if you don't want to be hurt, don't hurt someone else.

But no individual, in the prosecution of a typical drug offense, is ever identified as having been hurt. It is axiomatic that the drug user is preying on society–committing crimes, taking welfare, not paying taxes, ignoring the welfare of his children, driving stoned. This presumption underlies the retributive approach.

It is also axiomatic that the drug user (and, therefore, a criminal possessor of the drug) is hurt physically, mentally, emotionally and morally by the drug use. This presumption underlies an application of the restorative justice model to drug offenses.

In the popular and scientific worlds alike, "addiction is a disease" (Lindesmith, 1965). This is an article of faith among persons in recovery, educated in the precepts of the Twelve-Step programs of Narcotics Anonymous (Narcotics Anonymous, 1987, p. 3). This concept, as in "alcoholism is a disease," was originally developed by Dr. Benjamin Rush in 1784 (Sullum, 2003, pp. 72-74) and adopted by Alcoholics Anonymous as a metaphor for the loss of control. There are numerous drug-related dependency disorders for which there is a description in the *Diagnostic and Statistical Manual of Disorders* (DSM-IV) of the American Psychiatric Association. In marking the twenty-fifth anniversary of the National Institute on Drug Abuse (NIDA), Director Alan Leshner wrote, "Over the last quarter century, biological and behavioral research conducted by NIDA's intramural and extramural scientists has clearly shown that drug abuse is a preventable behavior and drug addiction is a treatable brain disease" (Leshner, 1999). One might reasonably conclude that a drug user needs treatment, not criminal prosecution.

All drug users are universally presumed to be harmed by their drug use and to be hurting others. First-time drug offenders are almost invariably considered candidates for treatment to rehabilitate them from the harms they suffer from their drug use, and to prevent further (if unspecified) harm to society. If they resist treatment or fail to complete the course of treatment as ordered by a court, then they are punished.

Repeat offenders are presumed to be the most harmed by drug use and to inflict the most harm on society. They are thus usually punished more severely for having failed prior courses of treatment or punishment (i.e., evidence of a more serious affliction with the disease).

Punishing the ill is inhumane; punishing the more seriously ill is barbaric. The punishment, always a loss of freedom and usually a term of imprisonment, compounds the hurt. Imprisonment, with an enormous psychological and social price, with heightened risk of exposure to infectious diseases, and exposure to inmate-on-inmate violence, usually exceeds the actual hurt caused by the illegal drug that is the occasion for the prosecution (Human Rights Watch, 1993; Forer, 1994, pp. 73-95).

Lost in the zeal of drug enforcement and the assembly line of the courts is the reality that drug users are ordinary citizens. Roughly three-quarters of current illegal drug users are employed full time or part time. While "alcoholism alone accounts for 500 million lost workdays each year" (White House, 2000a, p. 47), a typical consequence of a drug arrest and conviction is the loss of employment altogether.

In the course of prosecuting a drug possession offense, the prosecution, the court, the media, and even the defense counsel, presume the existence of harms inflicted by this drug user upon others. But the indictment never alleges these harms. Direct and indirect punishment that adds to the hurt experienced by the drug user is usually imposed without any evidence that the conduct being punished actually harmed anyone.

The hollowness of this presumption is revealed by the fact that there is almost never any effort to seek restitution for those who are presumed to have been harmed. In general, the retribution of drug possession prosecutions is disconnected from any infliction of harm to others by the defendant. Manski, Pepper and Petrie (2001) observe, "Sanctions against drug use are a preeminent feature of policy on illegal drugs, yet very little is known about the actual effects of these sanctions on drug use (independent of the effects of other social controls)" (2001, p. 188). However, there is a movement to provide the public the opportunity to sue participants in the drug market civilly under a model Drug Dealer Liability Act already adopted by fourteen states <http://www.modelddla.com/> (accessed Feb. 3, 2003).

The concept of restorative justice is a major reform of the misplaced focus on crime as an offense against the state in the offender-oriented retributive model of criminal justice. Following the impulse to heal the injured and society, a program or system of restorative justice sees the presumably injured drug offender and responds with treatment. In the simple restorative model, the justice system will be required to provide drug treatment instead of traditional punishment. The reduced loss of freedom and collateral consequences of arrest and conviction are accepted by reformers as a small price for the drug user offender to pay for such a humanizing improvement upon the retributive system. Vaillant (2001) argues that a combination of coercion and care can be effective in treating opiate addiction, following the careers of several cohorts of New York City heroin addicts. He notes that coercion does not simply mean criminal justice system control. The coercion can be voluntary, such as maintaining abstinence in order to remain employed while participating in an employee assistance program. A carrot and stick approach, not found in either the criminal justice or medical model, may be most successful.

Our drug policy is the antithesis of a restorative policy. Under the war on drugs, the death rate from illegal drug use has more than doubled in the past two decades. In 1979, 7,101 people died from drug abuse. In 1998, 20,227 people died from drug abuse. Proportionately, very few of them were minors. The drug-related death rate in 1979 was 3.2 per 100,000. In 1998, the death rate was 7.5 per 100,000 (White House, 2002a, table 20, p. 71). In the last decade the incidence of persons reporting drug use when being treated at hospital emergency departments has increased more than 60%, from 371,000 in 1990 to 602,000 in 2000 (White House, 2002a, table 21, p. 72), suggesting that drugs are more potent, more frequently contaminated with poisons, or that prevalence is increasing.

During the 1990s, high school seniors reported that they perceived illegal drugs to be more available to them than their predecessors had reported. By 1998 the perception of easy availability reached unprecedented rates: 35.6 percent of the high school class of 1998 reported that heroin was "fairly easy" or "very easy to get," more than any year since 1975 when the survey began; 90.4 percent of the high school class of 1998 reported that marijuana was "fairly easy" or "very easy to get," more than any year since 1975. Since then there has been a decline in perceived easy availability—down to 29.0 percent for heroin and to 87.2 percent for marijuana reported by the class of 2001 (Johnston, O'Malley, & Bachman, 2002, table 13).

Despite the avowal of Gen. Barry McCaffrey that the Federal antidrug program was expanding drug treatment capacity, the number of persons needing drug abuse treatment has not significantly declined (White House, 2001, table 42, p. 169).

Drug use by persons who commit crimes against persons or property is widespread. The Arrestee Drug Abuse Monitoring program (ADAM) reports for cities around the country a great range of positive urine samples for persons arrested for a variety of offenses. In most jurisdictions in 1997, for example, one-quarter to one-third of violent offenders tested positive for cocaine and one-quarter to one-half tested positive for marijuana. For property crime, there was a great deal of variation between cities in the percentage of arrestees with positive urinalyses for cocaine or marijuana—between twenty and sixty percent (ADAM, 1998).

Those who commit crimes against others must be differentiated from those who are convicted of only violating the controlled substances laws. Predatory offenders deserve an appropriate punishment and society should intervene to reduce the likelihood of re-offending. Given that many predatory offenders are not merely users of illegal drugs and alcohol but are highly dependent, one such intervention is in-prison drug treatment. Pellissier, Rhodes, Saylor, Gaes, Camp, Vanyur, and Wallace (2000) found that there were serious methodological problems in many of the evaluations of in-prison drug treatment programs, which generally claimed lower rates of recidivism. However, they found for the Federal Bureau of Prisons program that both male and female former prisoners, who had completed the BOP program, were somewhat less likely to be rearrested or to use drugs after three years, compared to those who did not participate in the program.

RETRIBUTION AGAINST TRAFFICKERS

The drug user has a mixed image: sympathetically a person with the disease of addiction, and unsympathetically a thoughtless neglecter of one's family or a predatory thief for money to buy drugs, etc. In contrast, with terrorists and child molesters, drug traffickers are an archetype of the menacing offender, e.g., the mythical school-yard drug pusher, hurting everyone and society at large. But the prosecution rarely offers evidence that any individual has been hurt by the acts of trafficking committed by the accused. (At a trial, or arguing against a reduction in bail, the prosecutor invariably refers to the horrible consequences to society of drug use and the drug trade, even though no facts on this point are entered into evidence.)

CRIMINAL JUSTICE SYSTEM PROBLEMS

American drug policy is a paradigmatically retributive policy. On September 1, 1973, new anti-drug laws took effect in New York State. These laws required mandatory minimum prison terms for persons convicted of selling drugs, even though Congress repealed the federal mandatory minimum sentences in the Controlled Substances Act of 1970 (P.L. 91-513, Oct. 27, 1970). The possession of one ounce, or the sale of two ounces, of heroin or cocaine, for example, now results in a prison sentence of at least fifteen years, with a maximum of life imprisonment. Parole from such sentence now results in lifetime supervision, unlike the termination of parole supervision of murder or lesser crimes, as soon as five years after release. For smaller quantities, or other drugs, there is a mandatory minimum of six years (Joint Committee on New York Drug Law Evaluation, 1977). Governor Nelson Rockefeller crusaded for these laws, in part to rebut the perception of him as a liberal–a great obstacle to winning the Republican presidential nomination (Epstein, 1990, p. 38). According to Szasz (1974), *The New York Times* (Feb. 12, 1973) quoted Gov. Rockefeller, "We, the citizens, are imprisoned by [drug] pushers. I want to put the pushers in prison so we can come out." At the end of 2002, an organization, Dads and Mad Moms Against Drug Dealers, was petitioning New York State legislators to toughen the Rockefeller drug laws, calling drug traffickers "parasites" <www.dammadd.org/Petition.pdf>.

Once a society accepts that some of its members are "parasites" there is no limit to the ostracism and punishment that can be justified. In

1986, without hearings, the Congress raised the maximum penalty for violating the federal Controlled Substances Act of 1970 from 20 years to life imprisonment (P.L. 99-570, sec. 1002).

Characterized as vermin, drug traffickers are worthy of extermination. On Sept. 25, 1996, Speaker of the U.S. House of Representatives Newt Gingrich (R-GA) introduced a bill, the Drug Importer Death Penalty Act of 1996, to impose the death penalty on a person who imported more than 100 doses of an illegal drug (for marijuana less than three ounces) after a conviction for drug importation (H.R. 4170, 105th Cong.). "If you sell it, we're going to kill you," he said (Abrams, 1997).

The American criminal justice system is now bedeviled by problems that flow from this system of controlling drugs. In the past twenty-five years there has been a diminution in the amount of due process afforded to an accused drug offender (Wisotsky, 1990, pp. 117-126).

Criminal court dockets are crowded with far more cases than can be properly and thoughtfully accommodated. The number of criminal cases filed per federal judge was substantially higher in the late 1990s compared to the early 1980s for 63 out of 91 districts. In 11 districts there was a decline, and in 17 districts, little change (Pastore & Maguire, 2000, table 1.69, pp. 64-66).

Prison overcrowding is aggravated by drug prohibition prosecutions. From 1974 to 1984, drug offenders made up between 25% to 30% of the federal prison population. From 1992 to the present, drug offenders have made up between 58% to 60% of the federal prison population. The total federal prison population grew from 23,566 in 1973 to 100,639 in 1997 (Pastore & Maguire, 2000, table 6.48, p. 519). The federal prison population at the beginning of 2003 is approximately 165,000 (Johnson, 2003).

About one-third of Americans believe police brutality occurs in their area according to a 1999 Gallup poll (www.gallup.com). Some of the public impression about police conduct is created by the depiction of the violence characteristic of drug raids and arrest. The execution of such raids is now a cliché of television news on the Fox television network and its syndicated program COPS. News media accompaniment of police raids was commonplace prior to 1999 (*Wilson* v. *Layne*, 526 U.S. 903, 1999). The door is battered down by screaming police assault teams that charge into the home terrorizing the suspects and their families, as the police ransack the premises to find guns, cash, and drugs (Skolnick & Fyfe, 1993, pp. 16, 108). Chermak (1994, p. 105) notes that some television reporters believe depictions of police drug raids have a deterrent effect on drug use.

Undercover narcotics enforcement requires the police and their informants to establish false identities and to lie to the citizenry, including the suspects. The questionable morality of such dishonesty undertaken by the state, and its consequences, were examined by Marx (1988). Such investigations often permit drug trafficking to be carried on as evidence is gathered and suspects are identified, undermining respect for the law (Marx, 1988, p. 97). A consequence of such professional deception is that even lying under oath is seen as permissible. Perjury by police officers in the enforcement of drug cases is endemic. Officers lie in their warrant applications, in their reports, in their debriefings to supervisors and prosecutors, and in their testimony (Gray, 2001, pp. 75, 111-112; Skonick & Fyfe, 1993, p. 35). Perjured testimony was commonplace in New York City, and known among the police as "testilying" (Sexton, 1994).

Racial discrimination in the justice system is exacerbated in drug enforcement. African-Americans, Africans, and Hispanics are stopped and searched at rates that exceed the rates at which white persons are stopped and searched in the hunt for drug offenders. Using race as a key factor in the decision to stop is known as racial profiling. Harris (2002) has found that racial profiling of people of color continues inexorably even though a number of studies show people of color are less likely to be carrying drugs (or weapons) than whites. Examining the hit rate in New Jersey, for example, the percentage of whites searched who have drugs is almost twice as high as the percentage of blacks (and five times the percentage of Hispanics) who have drugs (Harris, 2002, p. 80). The waste of law enforcement resources and labor, and the ineffectiveness of racial profiling, suggest that it endures to serve objectives unrelated to the detection of crime and the prosecution of offenders. One consequence of excessive focus on the interdiction of people of color is racial disparity in prosecution and punishment (Human Rights Watch, 2000).

THE EXTENT OF THE DRUG PHENOMENON IN THE CRIMINAL JUSTICE SYSTEM

One common characteristic of criminal offenders in the U.S. is that they are illegal drug users. Urinalysis of persons arrested for money-seeking street crime in major cities around the nation reveals evidence of recent use of illegal drugs at rates in the range of 51% to 80% of the arrestees (Taylor, Fitzgerald, Hunt, Reardon, & Brownstein, 2001). The general consensus of the research is that the career of offending preceded the career of illegal drug use (Chaiken & Chaiken, 1990). But illegal drug use is often an aspect of outlaw lifestyle and anti-social behavior (Faupel, 1991; Hanson, Beschner, Walters, & Bovelle, 1985).

One common characteristic of criminal justice agencies in the U.S. is the extensive focus on possession and distribution of illegal drugs. Nationwide, the category, drug offenses, is the largest of any crime reported in the annual reports of the nation's arrests (known as the Uniform Crime Reports) with 1,579,566 persons arrested in 2000. There are twice as many drug arrests in a year as there are arrests for all crimes of violence (FBI, 2001, p. 216). In 1994, 31.9 percent of new prison admissions were for drug offenses, more than for property offenses (31.3%) or violent crime (18.4%) (Maguire & Pastore, 1998, table 5.49, p. 424). Since 1992, drug offenders have comprised between 58% and 60% of the Federal prison population (Pastore & Maguire, 2000, table 6.48, p. 519).

The prohibited drug trade is a retail business with revenues of more than $60 billion annually (White House, 2002a, p. 57). This revenue is equal to the 13th largest corporation in the country, and greater than the 2001 revenues of AT&T, Boeing, or Bank of America (Fortune, 2002). The industry employs hundreds of thousands of persons. Over 300,000 persons were arrested for the prohibited manufacturing or trafficking in 2000 (FBI, 2001), a typical recent number, without any diminution in the supply of drugs, and without any increase in the retail price of drugs.

The prohibited drug trade creates and adds to disorder in low-income neighborhoods throughout the nation. Illegal drugs are very expensive (White House, 2002a, p. 81). Compulsive drug users operate in a cycle of expensive drug use and crime to pay for the drugs (Faupel, 1991).

CONSEQUENCES OF PHILOSOPHY
OF RETRIBUTION TOWARD DRUG USERS

Some fourteen million Americans in 2000 used illegal drugs (including inhalants such as gasoline); 7.2 million were 26 years old, or older, 4.6 million were 18 to 25, and 2.3 million were 12 to 17 years old. Three-quarters of the illegal drug users use marijuana, and 59% of illegal drug users use marijuana exclusively (SAMHSA, 2001, p. 13). The adult marijuana users live apparently normal lives (Zimmer & Morgan, 1997). These persons consider their use of marijuana and other drugs to be beneficial and pleasant (Gottlieb, 1987). For them, the physical or medical risks of injury are comparable to the risks of many other normal activities. American drug policy does not acknowledge any of the users' perceived benefits from using illegal drugs (White House, 2002a; Sterling, 1997a).

If traffickers can be characterized as parasites to be eradicated, how much more benign is the view of drug users? Since the early 1980s, DEA Administrators, for example, have advised Congress that America cannot "arrest its way out of the drug problem." The alternative is demand reduction. But this is not an innocent reframing of the problem as prevention, social reform, or education. Demand reduction has meant, in reality, solving the problem of the continued existence of drug users mainly through harsh punishment of them and their families. Miller (1996) draws a strong parallel between the labeling of the Jews in Germany as a social problem in the 1930s and their ever-increasing ostracism and exclusion from the economy and society, and the increasing social isolation of drug users in the United States by means of ever more elaborate legal sanctions.

In the late 1980s, Congress' anti-drug laws were designed to achieve a solution to the problem of drug users. The Anti-Drug Abuse Act of 1988 provided that any individual convicted for a Federal or state drug offense was to be ineligible for most Federal benefits (P.L. 100-690, sec. 5301). The Act also stated, "It is the declared policy of the United States Government to create a Drug-Free America by 1995," (P.L. 100-690, sec. 5251(b)). For responsible drug users, such language faintly echoes of a "final solution."

Recently, the U.S. Supreme Court upheld a provision of the Anti-Drug Abuse Act of 1988 (sec. 5101) permitting the eviction from public housing of the families of drug users (*Dep't. of Housing and Urban Development* v. *Rucker*, 535 U.S. 125; 122 S. Ct. 1230; 152 L. Ed. 2d 258; 2002 U.S. LEXIS 2144; 2002). Drug users, indeed persons suspected of using drugs, can be barred from visiting their parents if they live in a public housing project. The Supreme Court of Virginia concluded a man who had been ordered not to enter a public housing project could not be convicted of trespass for violating a public housing anti-drug ordinance when bringing diapers to his child because the ban upon entering formerly public street (turned over to the public housing agency to control nonresident entry) was so broad it violated First Amendment rights to expression in public places (*Commonwealth v. Hicks*, 264 Va. 48; 563 S. E. 2d 674; Va. 2002). However, the conviction was re-instated and the anti-drug ordinance was unanimously upheld by the U.S.

Supreme Court (*Virginia v. Hicks*, 539 U.S.–; 123 S. Ct. 219; 156 L. Ed. 2d 148; 2003 U.S. LEXIS 4782; 2003)

Congress permanently denied welfare (Temporary Assistance to Needy Families, or TANF) and food stamps to families when a parent has a felony drug conviction (although a state legislature may vote to opt out a state from such a denial) (P.L. 104-193, sec. 115; 42 U.S.C. 862a; August 22, 1996). And Congress denied Federal student loan aid to students with any drug convictions, even summary possession citations (P.L. 105-244, sec. 483(f); 20 U.S.C. 1091(r); October 7, 1998). None of these sanctions are applied to convicted murderers, rapists or child molesters.

A noncitizen convicted of any drug offense or regulation (other than one involving less than 30 grams of marijuana) must be barred from entry into the United States or deported from the United States, no matter when the offense took place (8 U.S.C. 1227(a)(2)(B)).

The right to vote upon a felony conviction is lost in most states. This penalty has spread through the population with the dramatic rise in drug prosecutions (Fellner & Mauer, 1998).

In drug policy, the retribution paradigm is blindly followed, even when lethal to thousands of persons. The Centers for Disease Control, the Public Health Service, the National Academy of Sciences, and the American Public Health Association have called for the distribution of sterile syringes to injection drug users to prevent the deadly spread of HIV and hepatitis (Normand, Vlahov, & Moses, 1995). But in order to avoid "sending the wrong message to youth" about drugs, the White House and the Congress refuse to fund such public health interventions (White House, 2001, pp. 56, 73). This intervention optimally would prevent 14,000 new HIV infections annually (Day, 2002, p. 11).

THE RETRIBUTIVE RATIONALE
FOR DRUG ENFORCEMENT

The retributive rationale for drug enforcement rests upon a logical and moral contradiction. Drug use must be prohibited because its use leads to involuntary use and the loss to addiction of a person's freedom. But a person who obtains and uses drugs–whether experimentally, to get "high" or even to maintain his addiction–is found to have sufficient voluntary intent to have broken the law, and thus should be deprived of his freedom and jailed. If he doesn't give up his illegal drug use, he should either be forced to submit to treatment or submit to imprisonment so that he won't use drugs, which take away his freedom to make rational choices.

Drug users are presumed to be incapable of free choice, and thus are not entitled to be treated as adults. This coercion is for their own good, and the good of society–even if it cannot be shown that the particular drug user is actually harming himself; even if it cannot be shown that the particular drug user is actually harming society; even if it *can* be shown that the prohibition policy is causing significant harms to society.

The social and political desire to stigmatize illegal drug users extends to the stigmatization of seriously ill medical patients who use marijuana with their physicians' knowledge and recommendation. The government insists that there is no medical benefit that can be found in marijuana (White House, 2001, p. 56). But there is significant medical value in the constituent chemicals of marijuana (Joy, Watson, & Benson, 1999). In 1999, the Institute of Medicine of the National Academy of Sciences concluded that there was no alternative to smoking cannabis for some persons with pain or AIDS wasting (Joy, Watson, & Benson, 1999, pp. 8, 179). Dale Gieringer estimates that there are now 30,000 patients using cannabis pursuant to their physician's recommendation in California (Haleakala Times, 2002).

Public understanding of drug users as suffering from a treatable disease has been growing. In 2000, Proposition 36 passed in California to require that drug treatment be provided to arrested drug users instead of incarceration. In 2002, the initiative's sponsor, the Campaign for New Drug Policies, planned similar initiatives in Michigan, Florida, Ohio and the District of Columbia, which were opposed by the White House drug czar, and the anti-drug establishment (Forbes, 2002). Beginning with the Super Bowl in January 2002 the White House has paid for television ads that say that teenage marijuana users are supporting bombing and assassinations by international terrorists. The ostensible goal of the advertising is to discourage drug use, but the underlying goal is to stigmatize drug users as the economic supporters of terrorists. This is designed to undermine public sympathy for drug users as persons needing treatment and not deserving punishment.

GROWTH OF THE RETRIBUTION AND CRIMINAL JUSTICE RESPONSE TO DRUG USE

Drug use was rampant among American military personnel serving in Vietnam, many of whom were African-American or Latino (Baum,

1997, pp. 48). It was feared that returning personnel, twenty percent of whom were reported to be addicted to heroin, would fuel a crime wave in the U.S. Having promised to fight crime in his 1968 campaign, and responding to the connections between drug use, drug trafficking and crime, President Richard Nixon declared war on drugs in 1971 (Terkel, 1997, p. 29). Nixon made expansion of heroin treatment a major priority before the 1972 elections (Massing, 1998). After the election, these initiatives were set aside by the distraction of the Watergate scandal investigation, and Nixon's resignation in 1974.

Nixon created several new retribution-oriented, enforcement entities. The Drug Enforcement Administration, created in 1973 in the Department of Justice, became permanent.

The contemporary war on drugs commenced with the demise of the Carter Administration's policy of marijuana decriminalization in 1978 (Baum, 1997, pp. 112-136; Musto, 1999, pp. 262-267). An uninterrupted increase in spending across government levels for anti-drug efforts has ensued (White House, 1991, 2000b).

In FY 2002, there were the equivalent of over 52,000 full-time employees in the federal government working in and in support of drug enforcement, including 18,630 in the Bureau of Prisons, 8,171 in the Drug Enforcement Administration, 6,987 in the U.S. Customs Service, 5,913 in the Judiciary, 4,948 in the U.S. Coast Guard, 3,684 in the Immigration and Naturalization Service, 3,221 in the FBI, 1,742 in the U.S. Attorneys Offices, 1,634 in the U.S. Marshals Service, and 1,092 in the Bureau of Alcohol, Tobacco and Firearms. At least eleven additional agencies employed enforcement or enforcement support personnel devoted to anti-drug programs. The FY 2002 enacted federal anti-drug budget was $18.8 billion (White House, 2002b). State and local drug enforcement spending was estimated at $33 billion in 1996 by ONDCP Director Barry McCaffrey as reported by Blumenson and Nilsen (1998, p. 37).

Since 1982, almost every Congress has passed anti-drug laws to crack down on drug dealers and drug users. An anti-drug, anti-crime package passed in December 1982 was vetoed by President Reagan because it provided for a cabinet-level drug czar who, the Attorney General feared, would interfere with his responsibilities (Gest, 2001, pp. 48-49). In 1984 Congress passed the Comprehensive Crime Control Act of 1984, which created a presumption in favor of pretrial detention of all defendants who are charged with a drug offense carrying a sentence of more than 10 years (notwithstanding the bail provision of the Eighth Amendment) (P.L. 98-473, sec. 203, creating 18 U.S.C. 3142(e)). This affects most federal drug defendants and the majority of federal drug offenses (21 U.S.C. 841 *et seq.*). New mandatory minimum sentences for drug offenses were also created in 1984 (Musto, 1999, pp. 273-274; P.L. 98-473, sec. 503, creating 21 U.S.C. 845A).

In 1986, in the Anti-Drug Abuse Act, Congress created many mandatory minimum prison sentences for drug offenses (P.L. 99-570, sec. 1002), notwithstanding Congress' repeal of drug mandatory minimums in 1970. In the Anti-Drug Abuse Act of 1988, the drug crimes of attempt and conspiracy were brought under the mandatory minimum sentence scheme, as well as simple possession of crack cocaine (P.L. 100-690, sec. 6470 and sec. 6371). This has resulted in the mushrooming of the Federal prison population described above.

RETRIBUTION DRUG POLICY WAS PROMOTED TO MAINTAIN WHITE PRIVILEGE

Racism can be understood as a struggle by members of one race to maintain their privileged status vis-á-vis people of another race (Wilkins, 2001, pp. 19-20). Most white persons–who are unfailingly polite to persons of other races, who would never knowingly discriminate against a person of another race–are the beneficiaries of white privilege.

After slavery, the Durkeimian "collective conscience" in favor of white privilege did not change.

It is useful to view the twentieth century phenomenon of drug control in America overlaid on the century's relations between whites and blacks. The century begins, legally, with the Supreme Court decision of *Plessy v. Ferguson* (163 U.S. 357 (1896)) approving "separate but equal" segregation, casting white privilege in legal concrete, and framing the status of the races for two-thirds of the century. Every decade until 1970 was marked by frequent outbreaks of white violence against blacks in a struggle to maintain white privilege in the face of African-American advancement (Franklin, 1967, pp. 439-444, 479; Kennedy, 1997, pp. 41-47).

The first comprehensive federal narcotics law, the Harrison Narcotics Act, having been defeated in 1910, was enacted in 1914 after a campaign explicitly revised to exploit racial slanders (Musto, 1999, pp. 43-44, 305, 319). To the Southern Democrats dominating Congress, the unwanted expansion of federal police power became palatable when sold as the response to accounts such as, "Most of the attacks upon white women of the South are the direct result of a cocaine-crazed Negro Brain" (Musto, 1999, p. 305).

During the "Great Depression" and the "Dust Bowl," white families had to compete for scarce jobs with Mexican-Americans and immigrants from Mexico. If demonized, persons of Mexican descent were at a disadvantage. White labor leaders, politicians and publishers created the narrative that Mexicans were marijuana users and marijuana use caused violence. The drive to maintain white privilege helped to outlaw marijuana (Musto, 1999, pp. 219-223; Bertram, Blachman, Sharpe, & Andreas, 1996, p. 80), leading to the jailing of over eleven million persons between 1965 and 1997 (Thomas, 1998).

THE MODERN ENTWINING OF RACIAL DISCRIMINATION AND THE WAR ON DRUGS

The 1960s and 1970s were marked by dramatic change in American society, especially the legal conclusion of the bloody, century-long Civil Rights struggle. This affected crime rates. As Blumstein and Wallman note,

> The marked growth in [general criminal] violence between 1965 and the early 1970s may have been, at least in part, a result of the decline in perceived legitimacy of American social and governmental authority during this turbulent period, which contained the civil rights movement and the strident opposition to the war in Vietnam. The continuing up trend from 1970 to 1980 and the decline to 1985 are largely attributable to the movement of the baby-boom generation into and then out of the high-crime ages of the late teens and early twenties . . . (Blumstein & Wallmann, 2000, p. 4)

Simultaneously, a large and powerful youth culture arose. Widespread use of marijuana and psychedelic drugs such as LSD were key parts of this "cultural revolution" (Gottlieb, 1987). Drug use among young people grew enormously (Baum, 1997, pp. 120-121; Musto, 1999, pp. 246-248).

In 1968, Richard M. Nixon ran for president pledging to restore "law and order"–a theme tailored to capture white votes. The theme was integral to his "Southern Strategy" to capture white voters who were abandoning the Democratic Party in the South because of its support of civil rights legislation (Epstein, 1990, pp. 60-62). And whites in the north were in shock after three years of urban riots by blacks (Baum, 1997, pp. 10-12).

It was during the Nixon Administration that a four-decade stable rate of incarceration, at about 110 per 100,000, came to an end (Blumstein & Cohen, 1973). What explains this remarkable correctional transformation? By 1970, the forty-year campaign of the NAACP Legal Defense and Education Fund had successfully ended legal segregation. Blumstein and Cohen in their important paper observed "punishment takes many forms in a society" (1973, p. 201). They focused on "deviant" behavior, punished by the criminal justice system and listed processes of the justice system as forms of punishment other than imprisonment. Focusing upon the criminal justice system, they did not take into account that the "collective conscience" in America for centuries has effectively seen as blacks as "deviant" *per se*. When black persons violated the codes of segregation, they were prosecuted or more frequently punished extrajudicially. But long-standing obedience to these codes was far more restricting, degrading, and punishing–indeed dehumanizing–than any kind of probation or community corrections. Blumstein and Cohen did not evaluate segregation as a form of punishment reserved for the "deviant" status of being black, and what its abolition might mean to imprisonment rates.

But if their theory is correct, with the elimination of segregation as punishment, substitute forms of punishment would be necessary to maintain the stability of the society's response to what it finds deviant or offensive. Blumstein and Cohen anticipated shifts in society's determination of what was deviant. Looking at rising serious crime rates (violent crime rising 84.2 percent between 1960 and 1970), they suggested that perhaps society would become more lenient toward "non-victim crimes" such as drug use (1973, p. 204). But they noted that arrests for narcotics offenses increased 740.6 percent between 1960 and 1970, and 575 percent between 1965 and 1970. They predicted an adaptative response to this increase in punishment would soon be less serious punishment. And indeed, the Controlled Substances Act of 1970 had reduced simple possession from a felony to a misdemeanor. They saw the experience of the 1960s with increasing punishment of drug use leading to a reduction in penalties in 1970 as an example confirming their theory (1973, p. 206). But in a mistaken prediction, Blumstein and Cohen foresaw an imminent leveling off or decline in crime rates. But this they noted, by the logic of their theory, would be followed by the calls for life imprisonment and mandatory minimum drug sentences, that in one instance became the Rockefeller drug laws of 1973. But if crime rates go up (as they did), "we can reasonably expect to see increasing pressure for the decriminalization of the victimless crimes," (1973) (which was the case: marijuana possession was decriminalized by eleven states by 1979 [Kleiman, 1992, p. 434]).

The process of changing punishments in this fashion they note is implicit, intricate, continuous and complex. Drug abuse was popularly understood as a black problem, and drug use was illegal. Drugs were an ideal vehicle for new ventures in punishment and social control to maintain white privilege. Nixon's chief of staff, H.R. Haldemann wrote in his diary, "[President Nixon] emphasized that you have to face the fact that the whole problem is really the blacks. The key is to devise a system that recognizes this while not appearing to" (Baum, 1997, p.13).

Nixon's war on drugs was not only a measure to reduce crime; but also a symbolic tool to demonstrate intolerance for cultural ferment, youth protest, and black protest. By 1985 the incarceration rate had climbed to 313, by 1992 it had climbed to 505; by 1999 it had climbed to 682 per 100,000 (Pastore & Maguire, 2000, table 6.19, p. 497). The rate of white male incarceration climbed from 528 in 1985, to 990 in 1997. The rate of black male incarceration grew from 3,544 in 1985, to 6,838 in 1997 (Pastore & Maguire, 2000, table 6.20, p. 497).

For the last thirty-five years, the Republican Party has fought for the support of whites in the South, as was widely discussed in December 2002 after U.S. Senator Trent Lott (R-MS), the Republican Senate leader, endorsed Strom Thurmond's 1948 pro-segregation, pro-lynching presidential campaign (Crespino, 2002). The South is now the base of Republican political power.

The year 1980 was potentially a breakthrough year for the Republican Party. Ronald Reagan had to recapture the South, lost by Gerald Ford to Jimmy Carter in 1976, a former Georgia governor. For his first campaign trip after winning the nomination, Reagan went to the Neshoba County Fair in Philadelphia, Mississippi, on August 3, 1980 (Kneeland, 1980). With a population of less than 25,000, Neshoba County was not the vote-rich venue of traditional campaign kick offs. In 1980, Philadelphia, MS, was known only for the nationally broadcast disappearance of three civil rights workers there in 1964. Their kidnapping and murder by county deputy sheriffs was the spark that led to passage of the 1964 Civil Rights Act (Branch, 1998). In his speech to a crowd "almost entirely of whites," Reagan said, "I believe in states' rights" (Kneeland,

1980). Since the eighteenth century, "states' rights" has been the credo of the white Southern resistance to Yankee anti-slavery agitation and to Federal constitutional guarantees of civil rights to blacks (Franklin, 1967). Reagan's speech was a prime example of the importance of white privilege as the "south pole" of the Republican political compass. Even more importantly, it was his expression of support for the legal structures that maintain white privilege.

RACIAL DEVASTATION OF THE WAR ON DRUGS

Reagan came to office freezing and cutting federal domestic spending (Walsh, 1981; UPI, 1981). His first deviation from this policy, having proposed cuts in federal law enforcement in 1981, was an escalation of the "war on drugs" in 1982. Three weeks before the mid-term congressional election, Reagan announced an enormous expansion of federal drug enforcement: hiring at least 1,200 investigators and prosecutors at an initial cost of $160 to $200 million, at a time when DEA's entire Special Agent force totaled just over 1,800 agents. More spending was requested to house 1,200 to 1,500 federal prisoners. DoJ official Rudolph Giuliani denied the plan had any political motivation (Thornton, 1982).

In 1983, Reagan sent to Congress the largest package of anti-crime legislation since 1970, the Comprehensive Crime Control Act. Passed in 1984, the Act raised drug trafficking penalties (P.L. 98-473, secs. 502-503).

By 1986, the use of cocaine by the upper middle class had become déclassé. The Administration's Caribbean drug interdiction program had nearly eliminated the maritime shipment of bulky marijuana from Colombia. Colombian smugglers switched to sending cocaine in aircraft that reached the American south in a matter of hours. Cocaine hydrochloride, the export product, when combined with baking soda and water, is easily cooked into crack cocaine (technically, cocaine base) on a stovetop or in a microwave oven. Crack is easily vaporized and inhaled for a rush experienced more quickly than snorting cocaine powder.

Certainly there was a *terrible* problem of crack abuse among African-Americans in the 1980s. But in 1991, 2.427 million whites reported lifetime use of crack compared to 990 thousand blacks (ADAMHA,

1992, pp. 38-39). The fact that there were a greater number of white crack users than black never entered the public consciousness.

In 1986, Congress and the news media exploited the powder cocaine death of black basketball star Len Bias to create a hysteria about black crack users and crack dealers, and pregnant black women destroying their babies while smoking crack.

Upon Bias' death, the Democrats attempted to preempt the Republican success in exploiting the public's fears about drugs. An auction house atmosphere in the Congress led to mandatory minimum penalties for importing or distributing relatively small quantities of drugs (Baum, 1997, pp. 228-230). The most infamous penalty was a mandatory prison term of five years (up to 40 years) for distributing five grams of crack cocaine or 500 grams of powder cocaine (cocaine hydrochloride), and a mandatory term of ten years (up to life imprisonment) for distributing 50 grams of crack cocaine or 5,000 grams of powder cocaine (P.L. 99-570, Oct. 27, 1986, sec. 1002). Debate over the Anti-Drug Abuse Act of 1986 was media and political fodder from July 1986 to Election Day. It must be conceded that a number of black members of Congress called for action against crack and sponsored tough anti-crack bills. A majority of the black members of the House of Representatives voted for the Act (Kennedy, 1997, p. 370).

Within a few years, it appeared that blacks were being disproportionately sentenced for the crack cocaine offense. Congress called upon the U.S. Sentencing Commission to study the impact of mandatory minimum sentences (P.L.101-647, Nov. 29, 1990, Sec. 1703). The Commission found that the disparity in sentencing harshness between white and black offenders had increased (U.S. Sentencing Commission, 1991, p. 82). Congress and the Administration did nothing to address this problem.

By 1995, no white person had been prosecuted in federal court under the 1986 crack mandatory minimums in Los Angeles and other major cities, although hundreds of blacks had been (Weikel, 1995). Another study by the U.S. Sentencing Commission (1995) found the 100-to-1 powder cocaine-crack cocaine variation seemed to have an invidious impact on black offenders. For example, 88.3 percent of the mandatory crack sentences were imposed on blacks in FY 1993. The Commission recommended changes in the guidelines (60 Fed. Reg. 25,074, May 10, 1995), but for the first time Congress voted to disapprove the Commission's proposed amendments to the sentencing guidelines (P.L. 104-38, Oct. 30, 1995).

Through the 1970s, white juvenile drug offenders outnumbered blacks but this switched by the 1980s (Snyder & Sickmund, 1995, p. 120). Even though drug and alcohol use by black youth (except for marijuana) is one-half to one-quarter the rates of use by white youth (White House, 2002a, p. 63), the black juvenile drug arrest rate is five times the white juvenile drug arrest rate (Snyder & Sickmund, 1995, p. 120).

In fiscal year 2001, only one in four new federal drug prisoners was white (U.S. Sentencing Commission, 2002, table 34, p. 69). In 1997, for all offenses, only one in four new prisoners, nationwide, was white (Pastore & Maguire, 2000, table 6.17, p. 496). In 1996, 53% of all those convicted in state courts of a drug offense were black (Pastore & Maguire, 2000, table 5.50, p. 454)–even though only 38.4% of those arrested for a drug offense that year were black (FBI, 1997). *In 1999, sixty-five percent of all black federal prisoners were serving drug sentences* (Pastore & Maguire, 2000, table 6.47, p. 519). In 1998, the average federal drug sentence was 61.8 months for white prisoners and 109.8 months for black prisoners (Pastore & Maguire, 2000, p. 427).

Black people have been disproportionately stopped and searched, arrested, convicted, and imprisoned for drug offenses. Blacks are imprisoned for drug offenses at a rate that is 8.3 times greater than the rate of white imprisonment for drug offenses (Human Rights Watch, 2000). Thus to an utterly disproportionate and unjustifiable degree blacks are denied employment, housing, credit, college admissions, college loans, and the opportunity to travel. Indeed, African-Americans are strong supporters of the current drug laws–largely because the disorder of the drug trade is concentrated in their neighborhoods in most parts of the country. Reagan's 1982 initiative, his legislative priorities, his shaping of the public debate, and his Justice Department practices, carried forward by George H. W. Bush and Bill Clinton, made the war on drugs probably the most powerful instrument to maintain white privilege over the past twenty years.

Are most of those carrying out today's war on drugs deliberately racist? Certainly not. Certainly black communities continue to demand drug and law enforcement, which historically they have not received. But those in the criminal justice system are carrying out policies that have the effect of maintaining white privilege.

The war on drugs could only have been born in 1914 by exploiting white fears and revulsion at (false) stereotypes of blacks as drug-taking sex fiends and violent monsters. That paradigm was repeated throughout the twentieth century in the periods of drug war escalation. Curiously, the public overwhelmingly sees the war on drugs as failing (Kohut, 2001). Yet this policy persists because the white majority believes it protects them from drug trafficking blacks, Latinos and Asians. If whites were being stopped, searched, arrested, convicted, imprisoned and denied jobs, housing, credit, and voting rights because of drug offenses, at the *rates* blacks are, calls for ending the war on drugs would echo throughout the land.

POLITICALLY ACCEPTABLE ALTERNATIVES TO THE "WAR ON DRUGS"

One response to this history of failure and imprisonment is to urge that the anti-drug effort be redirected to treatment and prevention. Unfortunately, these dimensions actually offer little prospect of ameliorating the problems outlined above.

The conventional wisdom is that we need more treatment to solve the drug abuse problem. Of course, treatment means abstinence. RAND's Rydell and Everingham (1994) showed that cocaine treatment was far more cost effective than source country control, interdiction or domestic enforcement (imprisonment) policies in reducing consumption of cocaine. But using their model, even if drug treatment were to be given to every heavy user of cocaine every year, the total consumption of cocaine would be reduced, after 15 years, by only about one-third (Rydell & Everingham, 1994, p. 47). Treatment is humane and cost-effective, and it can help manage and reduce the harms (Bertram, Blachman, Sharpe, & Andreas, 1996, p. 212). But it will not rid the criminal justice system of the burden of drug cases, nor will it end the racial disparity of drug enforcement.

The other liberal hope, drug abuse prevention, is also doubtful as a solution (MacCoun & Reuter, 2001, p. 407). Despite Congress' repeated votes for effective drug abuse prevention, nationally, drug abuse prevention has been a failure. For over a decade, evaluators have repeatedly found that the nation's largest drug abuse prevention program, D.A.R.E. (Drug Abuse Resistance Education) is ineffective (Kanoff, 2003). Yet D.A.R.E. is the drug prevention program found in 80 percent of America's school districts, and is specifically written into the Federal drug abuse prevention legislation (20 U.S.C. 7116(b)(9)). In fact, the

Substance Abuse and Mental Health Services Administration identified only 41 effective school-based drug abuse prevention programs out of 718 evaluated (Kanoff, 2003). Effective programs have remained a tiny part of the nation's anti-drug effort even though they have been identified since the 1980s (Falco, 1992, pp. 36-38; Drug Strategies, 1999).

A NEW DRUG POLICY?

Instead of a war on drugs, I have advocated the management of the drug problem (Sterling, 1989; 1995; 1998). We don't call for a pollution-free America, even though air and water pollution lead to cancer and pulmonary disease. We manage those problems by regulating poisonous discharges from automobiles, businesses, and sewage treatment plants.

The economic, legal and political complexity of managing those problems is a clue to what must replace the simple (and simple-minded) approach of drug prohibition. But drug policy cannot be revised independently of refocusing our criminal justice and correctional systems (Sterling, 1998, pp. 499-502).

Lindesmith (1965) argued that the care of drug addicts, especially opiate addicts, be placed in the care of private physicians, and no longer handled as a police problem (pp. 270-273). Nadelmann (1992) in arguing for drug legalization suggests that most drug users engage in rational drug consumption. He argues "legal availability does not always connote easy availability and that restricted legal status of a drug does not always make it that difficult to obtain" (p. 109). He claims a "right of access" for adults that include a "right to possess small amounts of any drug for personal consumption" and "the right to obtain any drug from a reliable, legally regulated source." This source could be mail order, which could preclude the easy, impulsive availability of a local retail outlet, and would eliminate the role of physician as "gatekeeper." I have also argued that there is a right to use drugs, grounded in the First Amendment (Sterling, 1997a).

But the discussion of drug policy has suffered from a lack of clarity in the use of terms such as legalization. Nadelmann (1992) explicitly notes that he uses the term in a variety of ways (p. 87). I have attempted to identify these meanings and clarify terms such as "medicalization" as used by former Baltimore Mayor Kurt Schmoke, and "decriminalization" as used by the Shafer Commission (1973) (Sterling, 1995, pp. 399-406).

Drug use is too harmful to prohibit, or to legalize without controls. Only regulation of drug distribution and use can manage the problem to reduce the harms. Alcohol, estimated to cause in excess of 100,000 deaths per year, for example, is considered legal. But, without special federal, state and local licenses, most people cannot manufacture or distribute alcohol (except for small scale home brewing and wine making).

Beer, wine and whiskey are simply three forms of the same drug, yet throughout the nation, they are taxed and regulated differently. Including zoning laws, restaurant laws, restrictions on advertising, time of day restrictions, restrictions on Sunday and Election Day sales, legal alcohol is extensively regulated. Such regulations are designed to minimize alcohol abuse, to eliminate crime in the distribution of alcohol, and to raise revenue–goals that are in obvious tension.

However, proposals to regulate drugs, i.e., to legalize them, are frequently mocked as selling crack in the supermarket (even though crack is illegally sold outside many supermarkets today). But it must be acknowledged that proposals to legalize drugs have usually lacked any specificity although Neustadter (1998) has collected and analyzed those that attempt specificity.

MacCoun and Reuter (2001) have identified the different types of controls. Between pure prohibition (e.g., heroin and LSD today) and a free market (e.g., caffeine–available without restriction to children and adults), they find roughly seven intermediate forms of drug control: prohibitory prescription allowing narrow therapeutic uses (e.g., cocaine); maintenance, such as methadone or the Swiss heroin maintenance experiment; regulatory prescription (self-administered under prescription); positive license (available to any licensed adult with demonstration of capacity for safe use); negative license (available to any licensed adult who has not forfeited the privilege by some transgression); availability to any adult (e.g., alcohol); and depenalization (elimination of criminal sanctions for possession, but sale and manufacture remain illegal) (pp. 74, 311).

The principal challenge in making or fairly reviewing any proposal is to balance the inevitable harms that will result or will remain against the reductions in harms that are sought to be reduced or eliminated. This is extraordinarily difficult, but MacCoun and Reuter (2001) have written the most sophisticated critique of current drug policy, the debate around drug legalization, and various possible alternatives to prohibition, which significantly influences my conclusion.

CONCLUSION

Any recommendation (and adoption) of a new policy must be tentative, and offered with great humility. It is truly impossible to predict with much precision how the complex market of drug users and traffickers will respond. Even the nation's most sophisticated consumer market specialists usually fail to predict the success of new offerings.

There is also no agreement on what is relevant evidence, the standards for judging it, and the placement of the burden of proof in either defending the status quo or offering a new control regime. Ultimately this will continue to sharpen as a political struggle.

Marijuana should be depenalized. Adults ought to be able to use it privately. They ought to be able to use it in their own homes, and in licensed premises and outdoors with the requirement that unconsenting persons must not be forced to inhale the smoke. They ought to be able to grow their own supply and to give it away without consideration. Parents ought to be able to initiate their teenagers in appropriate, responsible marijuana use, as they do with alcohol. A commercial distribution system, at this point, opens up the problems of advertising and promotion of use. During the 1990s I distributed a mock U.S. Treasury marijuana users license for a $100 per year annual fee, $200 to cultivate for one's own use (Sterling, 1998, pp. 511, 525). The case for depenalization seems compelling (MacCoun & Reuter, 2001, p. 362).

Heroin and other opiates should also be depenalized. The drugs should be available through physicians and consulting pharmacists. This is sometimes referred to as medicalization.

Hallucinogens have value and should be available from licensed leaders and to persons who are licensed to use the drugs (Sterling, 1997b). With professional licensing and a requirement of insurance to use or distribute these drugs, public and private regulatory bodies and private insurance market can develop standards to minimize risks of harm and costs.

It is premature to propose a regulated scheme to distribute cocaine and amphetamines. From a purely drug policy standpoint it would be sufficient now to make the other changes and study the evolving markets and patterns of use. But we must address the problem of cocaine illegality for "the minority poor that bear a disproportionate share of the harms of prohibition" (MacCoun & Reuter, 2001, p. 335). Penalties should be reduced. Cocaine trafficking or use infractions should not be *per se* bars to housing, credit, employment or public benefits.

The Controlled Substances Act is an oxymoron. There are no substances more out of control in our society or economy than the prohibited "controlled substances." The criminal justice system is one part of the regulatory structure of the environmental laws, the securities laws, and the antitrust laws. Criminal justice practitioners and theorists need to demand a reform of the drug laws to create genuine regulation and control.

REFERENCES

Abrams, J. (1997, May 8). Gingrich's Objectives. *Associated Press Wire*.

ADAM, Arrestee Drug Abuse Monitoring Program. (1998). *1997 Annual Report on Adult and Juvenile Arrestees*. Washington: National Institute of Justice.

ADAMHA, Alcohol, Drug Abuse and Mental Health Administration. (1992). *National Household Survey on Drug Abuse: Population Estimates 1991*. Rockville, MD: National Institute on Drug Abuse.

Baum, D. (1997). *Smoke and Mirrors: The War on Drugs and the Politics of Failure*. Boston: Little, Brown.

Bertram, E., Blachman, M., Sharpe, K., & Andreas, P. (1996). *Drug War Politics: The Price of Denial*. Berkeley, CA: University of California Press.

Blumenson, E. & Nilsen, E. (1998). Policing for Profit: The Drug War's Hidden Economic Agenda. *University of Chicago Law Review, 65, 35-114*.

Blumstein, A. & Cohen, J. (1973). A Theory of the Stability of Punishment. *Journal of Criminal Law & Criminology, 64, 198-207*.

Blumstein, A. & Wallman, J. (2000). *The Crime Drop in America*. New York: Cambridge University Press.

Branch, T. (1998). *Pillar of Fire: America in the King Years, 1963 65*. New York: Simon & Schuster.

Chaiken, J.M. & Chaiken, M.R. (1990). Drugs and Predatory Crime. In Tonry, M. & Wilson, J.Q. (Eds.), *Drugs and Crime* (pp. 203-239). Chicago, IL: University of Chicago Press.

Chermak, S. (1994). Crime in the News Media: A Refined Understanding of How Crimes Become News. In Barak, G. (Ed.), *Media, Process, and the Social Construction of Crime* (pp. 95-129). New York: Garland Publishing.

Crespino, J. (2002, Dec. 13). The Ways Republicans Talk About Race. *The New York Times*.

Day, D. (2002). *Health Emergency 2003: The Spread of Drug-Related AIDS and Hepatitis C Among African Americans and Latinos*. Princeton, NJ: The Dogwood Center.

Drug Strategies. (1999). *Making the Grade: A Guide to School Drug Prevention Programs*. Washington: Drug Strategies.

Epstein, E.J. (1990). *Agency of Fear: Opiates and Political Power in America.* (Rev'd Ed.). New York: Verso.

Falco, M. (1992). *The Making of a Drug-Free America: Programs that Work.* New York: Times Books.

Faupel, C.E. (1991). *Shooting Dope: Career Patterns of Hard-Core Heroin Users.* Gainesville, FL: University of Florida Press.

FBI. (1997). *Crime in the United States, 1996.* Washington: U.S. Government Printing Office.

FBI. (2001). *Crime in the United States, 2000.* Washington: U.S. Government Printing Office.

Fellner, J. & Mauer, M. (1998). *Losing the Vote: The Impact of Felony Disenfranchisement Laws in the United States.* Washington: The Sentencing Project and Human Rights Watch.

Forbes, D. (2002). *The Governor's Sub-rosa Plot to Subvert an Election in Ohio.* Washington: Institute for Policy Studies. <http://www.ips-dc.org/projects/drugpolicy/ohio.htm> (accessed Feb. 3, 2003).

Forer, L.G. (1994). *A Rage to Punish.* New York: W.W. Norton & Co.

Fortune Magazine. (2002). "America's Largest Corporations." <http://www.fortune.com/lists/F500/> (accessed Feb. 3, 2003).

Franklin, J.H. (1967). *From Slavery to Freedom: A History of Negro Americans,* 3rd Ed. New York: Alfred A. Knopf.

Gest, T. (2001). *Crime & Politics: Big Government's Erratic Campaign for Law and Order.* New York: Oxford University Press.

Goode, E. (1999). *Drugs in American Society, Fifth Edition.* New York: McGraw-Hill.

Gottleib, A. (1987). *Do You Believe in Magic? The Second Coming of the 60's Generation.* New York: Times Books.

Gray, J.P. (2001). *Why Our Drug Laws Have Failed and What We Can Do About It.* Philadelphia: Temple University Press.

Haleakala (HI) Times. (2002, Sept. 4). 30,000 Californians Using Medicinal Marijuana Legally.

Hanson, B., Beschner, G., Walters, J.M., & Bovelle, E. (1985). *Life with Heroin: Voices from the Inner City.* Lexington, MA: Lexington/D.C. Heath.

Harris, D.A. (2002). *Profiles in Injustice.* New York: W.W. Norton & Co.

Higginbotham, A.L., Jr. (1996). *Shades of Freedom: Racial Politics and Presumptions of the American Legal Process.* New York: Oxford University Press.

Human Rights Watch. (1993). *The Human Rights Watch Global Report on Prisons.* New York: Human Rights Watch.

Human Rights Watch. (2000, May). United States–*Punishment and Prejudice: Racial Disparities in the War on Drugs.* New York: Human Rights Watch. <http://www.hrw.org/reports/2000/usa/> (accessed Feb. 3, 2003).

Johnson, K. (2003, Jan. 23). Federal prisons are packed with almost 165,000. *USA Today.*

Johnston, L.D., O'Malley, P.M., & Bachman, J.G. (2002). *Monitoring the Future: National Survey Results on Drug Use, 1975-2001. Volume I. Secondary school students.* Bethesda, MD: National Institute on Drug Abuse.

Joint Committee on New York Drug Law Evaluation. (1977). *The Nation's Toughest Drug Law: Evaluating the New York Experience.* New York: Association of the Bar of the City of New York.

Joy, J.E., Watson, S.J., Jr., & Benson, J.A., Jr. (1999). *Marijuana and Medicine: Assessing the Science Base.* Washington: National Academy Press.

Kanoff, M.E. (2003). *Youth Illicit Drug Use Prevention: DARE Long-Term Evaluations and Federal Efforts to Identify Effective Programs.* Washington: General Accounting Office.

Kennedy, R. (1997). *Race, Crime, and the Law.* New York: Pantheon Books.

Kleiman, M.A.R. (1992). *Against Excess: Drug Policy for Results.* New York: Basic Books Harper Collins.

Kneeland, D.E. (1980, Aug. 4). Reagan Campaigns at Mississippi Fair. *New York Times,* p. A11.

Kohut, A. (2001, March 21). *The War on Drugs: Do the American People Have Battle Fatigue?* Washington: Center for National Policy.

Leshner, A.I. (1999, April). The Next Generation of Drug Abuse Research in *NIDA Notes* 14:1, 3. Bethesda, MD: National Institutes of Health, National Institute on Drug Abuse.

Lindesmith, A.R. (1965). *The Addict and the Law.* New York: Vintage/Random House.

Lusane, C. (1991). Pipe Dream Blues: Racism and the War on Drugs. Boston: South End Press.

MacCoun, R.J. & Reuter, P. (2001). *Drug War Heresies: Learning from Other Vices, Times, and Places.* New York: Cambridge University Press.

Maguire, K. & Pastore, A.L. (1998). *Sourcebook of Criminal Justice Statistics 1997.* Washington: Government Printing Office.

Manski, C.F., Pepper, J.V., & Petrie, C.V. (2001). *Informing America's Policy on Illegal Drugs: What We Don't Know Keeps Hurting Us.* Washington: National Academy Press.

Marx, G.T. (1988). *Undercover: Police Surveillance in America.* Berkeley, CA: University of California Press.

Massing, M. (1998). *The Fix.* New York: Simon & Schuster.

Miller, R.L. (1996). *Drug Warriors & Their Prey: From Police Power to Police State.* Westport, CT: Praeger.

Moore, M.H. (2001). Toward a Balanced Drug-Prevention Strategy: A Conceptual Map. In Heymann, P.B. & Brownsberger, W.N. (Eds.), *Drug Addiction and Drug Policy.* Cambridge, MA: Harvard University Press.

Musto, D. (1999). *The American Disease, Origins of Narcotic Control,* 3rd Ed. New York: Oxford University Press.

Nadelmann, E.A. (1992). Thinking Seriously About Alternatives to Prohibition. *Daedalus* 121, 85-132.

Narcotics Anonymous. (1987). *Narcotics Anonymous, Fourth Ed.* Van Nuys, CA: Narcotics Anonymous World Service Office.

Neustadter, S. (1998). Legalization Legislation: Confronting the Details of Policy Choices. In Fish, J.M. (Ed.), *How to Legalize Drugs.* Northvale, NJ: Jason Aronson, Inc.

Normand, J., Vlahov, D., & Moses, L.E. (1995). *Preventing HIV Transmission: The Role of Sterile Needles and Bleach*. Washington: National Academy Press.

Pastore, A.L. & Maguire, K. (Eds.). (2000). *Sourcebook of Criminal Justice Statistics-1999*. Washington: Bureau of Criminal Justice Statistics, U.S. Department of Justice.

Pellissier, B., Rhodes, W., Saylor, W., Gaes, G., Camp, S.D., Vanyur, S.D., & Wallace, S. (2000). *Triad Drug Treatment Evaluation Project Final Report of Three-Year Outcomes: Part 1*. Washington: Federal Bureau of Prisons, Office of Research and Evaluation.

Ray, O. & Ksir, C. (1999). *Drugs, Society and Human Behavior*. New York: WCB/McGraw Hill.

Rydell, C.P. & Everingham, S.S. (1994). *Controlling Cocaine: Supply versus Demand Programs*. Santa Monica, CA: RAND Drug Policy Research Center.

SAMHSA (Substance Abuse and Mental Health Services Administration). (2001). *Summary of Findings from the 2000 National Household Survey on Drug Abuse*. Rockville, MD: SAMHSA.

Sexton, J. (1994, April 22). New York Police Often Lie Under Oath, Report Says. *New York Times*.

Shafer, R.P. (1973). *Drug Use in America: Problem in Perspective; Second Report of the National Commission on Marihuana and Drug Abuse*. Washington: Government Printing Office.

Skolnick, J.H. & Fyfe, J.J. (1993). *Above the Law: Police and the Excessive Use of Force*. New York: Free Press.

Snyder, H.N. & Sickmund, M. (1995). *Juvenile Offenders and Victims: A National Report*, Washington: Office of Juvenile Justice and Delinquency Prevention.

Sterling, E.E. (1989, Sept. 30). Harm management, not drug-free nation, should become USA's anti-drug objective. *Law Enforcement News*. New York: John Jay College of Criminal Justice/CUNY.

Sterling, E.E. (1995). The Sentencing Boomerang: Drug Prohibition Politics and Reform. *Villanova Law Review*, 40, 383-427.

Sterling, E.E. (1997a). Drug Policy: A Smorgasbord of Conundrums Spiced by Emotions Around Children and Violence. *Valparaiso University Law Review*, 31, 597-645.

Sterling, E.E. (1997b). Law Enforcement Against Entheogens: Is it Religious Persecution? In R. Forte (Ed.), *Entheogens and the Future of Religion* (pp. 165-170). San Francisco: Council on Spiritual Practices.

Sterling, E.E. (1998). Principles and Proposals for Managing the Drug Problem. In Fish, J.M. (Ed.), *How to Legalize Drugs*. Northvale, NJ: Jason Aronson, Inc.

Sullum, J. (2003). *Saying Yes: In Defense of Drug Use*. New York: Teacher/Putnam.

Szasz, T. (1974). *Ceremonial Chemistry: The Ritual Persecution of Drugs, Addicts, and Pushers*. Garden City, New York: Anchor Press/Doubleday.

Taylor, B.G., Fitzgerald, N., Hunt, D., Reardon, J.A., & Brownstein, H.H. (2001). *ADAM Preliminary 2000 Findings on Drug Use and Drug Markets–Adult Male Arrestees*. Washington: National Institute of Justice.

Terkel, S.N. (1997). *The Drug Laws: A Time for Change?* New York: Franklin Watts.

Thomas, C. (1998). *Marijuana Arrests and Incarceration in the United States: Preliminary Report*. Washington: Marijuana Policy Project.

Thornton, M. (1982, Oct. 15). U.S. Escalates Newest War on Crime, Drugs. *Washington Post.*

United Press International. (1981, Mar. 23). Stockman Asserts that Administration Needs More than $40 Billion in Cuts. *Washington Post.*

United States Sentencing Commission. (1991). *Special Report to Congress: Mandatory Minimum Penalties in the Federal Criminal Justice System.* Washington: U.S. Sentencing Commission.

United States Sentencing Commission. (1995). *Special Report to the Congress: Cocaine and Federal Sentencing Policy.* Washington: U.S. Sentencing Commission.

United States Sentencing Commission. (2002). *2001 Sourcebook of Federal Sentencing Statistics.* Washington: U.S. Sentencing Commission.

Vaillant, G.E. (2001). If Addiction Is Involuntary, How Can Punishment Help? In Heymann, P.B. & Brownsberger, W.N. (Eds.), *Drug Addiction and Drug Policy.* Cambridge, MA: Harvard University Press.

Walsh, E. (1981, Mar. 7). Federal Spending Freeze Began Before Request Went to Congress. *Washington Post.*

Weikel, D. (1995, May 21). War on Crack Targets Minorities Over Whites. *Los Angeles Times.*

White House. (1991). *The National Drug Control Strategy: Budget Summary, February 1991.* Washington: U.S. Government Printing Office.

White House. (2000a). *The National Drug Control Strategy: 2000 Annual Report.* Washington: U.S. Government Printing Office.

White House. (2000b). *The National Drug Control Strategy: 2000 Annual Report, FY 2001 Budget Summary.* Washington: U.S. Government Printing Office.

White House. (2001). *The National Drug Control Strategy: 2001 Annual Report.* Washington: U.S. Government Printing Office.

White House. (2002a). *National Drug Control Strategy, February 2002.* Washington: U.S. Government Printing Office.

White House. (2002b). *National Drug Control Strategy, FY 2003 Budget Summary.* Washington: U.S. Government Printing Office.

Wilkins, R. (2001). *Jefferson's Pillow: The Founding Fathers and the Dilemma of Black Patriotism.* Boston: Beacon Press.

Wisotsky, S. (1990). *Beyond the War on Drugs.* Buffalo, New York: Prometheus Books.

Zimmer, L. & Morgan, J.P. (1997). *Marijuana Myths, Marijuana Facts.* New York: Lindesmith Center.

From Destruction to Reconciliation: The Potential of Restorative Justice

Daniel Johnson

SUMMARY. Daniel Johnson discusses how the application of "restorative justice" in his own life and in the life of the victim of his criminal offense contributed to his personal regeneration and healing for his victim. Mr. Johnson challenges criminal justice policy-makers to create conditions where "restorative justice" can be employed in the broadest sense in order to do what contemporary, punitive, retributive criminal justice systems are largely incapable of doing, that is, facilitate lasting offender rehabilitation and healing for crime victims and communities, and to offer opportunities for victim-offender reconciliations. *[Article copies available for a fee from The Haworth Document Delivery Service: 1-800-HAWORTH. E-mail address: <docdelivery@haworthpress.com> Website: <http://www.HaworthPress.com> © 2004 by The Haworth Press, Inc. All rights reserved.]*

Daniel Johnson has been incarcerated in the Texas prison system since 1977 because of a felony conviction for a sexual assault offense, his first felony conviction. He holds a BS degree in education, and held professional licenses as an insurance broker in real estate, and as a National Association of Security Dealer. He worked as an industrial engineer, schoolteacher, in sales and marketing, and as an independent businessman. He is a member of the board of advisors of Citizens United for the Rehabilitation of Errants (CURE).

Address correspondence to: Daniel Johnson, #274157, Post Office Box 15, Lovelady, TX 75851.

[Haworth co-indexing entry note]: "From Destruction to Reconciliation: The Potential of Restorative Justice." Johnson, Daniel. Co-published simultaneously in *Journal of Religion & Spirituality in Social Work* (The Haworth Social Work Practice Press, an imprint of The Haworth Press, Inc.) Vol. 23, No. 1/2, 2004, pp. 83-91; and: *Criminal Justice: Retribution vs. Restoration* (ed: Eleanor Hannon Judah, and Rev. Michael Bryant) The Haworth Social Work Practice Press, an imprint of The Haworth Press, Inc., 2004, pp. 83-91. Single or multiple copies of this article are available for a fee from The Haworth Document Delivery Service [1-800-HAWORTH, 9:00 a.m. - 5:00 p.m. (EST). E-mail address: docdelivery@haworth press.com].

http://www.haworthpress.com/web/JRSSW
© 2004 by The Haworth Press, Inc. All rights reserved.
Digital Object Identifier: 10.1300/J377v23n01_05

KEYWORDS. Texas, inmate, rehabilitation, victim services, therapy, victim healing, offender regeneration, forgiveness, reconciliation, challenge to policy-makers

I have been continuously imprisoned in the Texas prison system for over a quarter of a century, as punishment for a felony conviction for a sexual assault I committed against a woman in Houston, Texas. This has been my first time in prison, my first conviction. I had little knowledge of criminal justice matters during the mid 1970s and I harbored many of the misconceptions about criminal justice that are still prevalent today, and unfortunately continue to shape criminal justice policies. Criminal justice issues are generally morally messy because they focus on prisoners–a group of people with little political clout and little claim to compassion. In 1977 I entered the notoriously harsh Texas prison system, where prisoners who sincerely desired to regenerate themselves had to do so in spite of the prison system, not because of it.

During the course of my imprisonment I have participated in a number of worthwhile programs and activities that slowly took root in the Texas prison system. These include a volunteer group therapy program for sex offenders facilitated by psychologists, faith-based programs and initiatives, and communication with outside organizations, state and federal officials, on the subjects of treatment for sex offenders and improving prison conditions. I have testified before a Texas legislative panel on the subject of reducing recidivism and in a federal court proceeding, which involved an extensive overhaul of unconstitutional conditions of confinement in Texas prisons. Before I came to prison I had no idea that conditions of confinement could be so oppressive and counter-productive to a prisoner's rehabilitative efforts.

The defining point of my journey to personal regeneration came during January of 2002 as the result of an expanding program facilitated by the victims services division of the prison agency–a program I was not even aware of until a few months prior to January. It is called the "victim-offender dialogue" program. Through this program, in which a dialogue request is initiated by a victim of a criminal offense, I was given the opportunity to personally meet with the victim of my 1977 offense, the offense for which I remain imprisoned. It was one of the most profound, meaningful experiences of a lifetime.

During my regeneration process I had confronted the darkest truths about myself, and it was not easy. Through my own self-study efforts and group therapy sessions I learned that a deviant impulse is far from unexplainable. To facilitate my own healing I had to first recognize and deal with what it was in my own life that led me to offend. Over a period of time I felt that I had reached a point where I understood the cognitive distortions that I had developed during the time frame of my life when I offended. With the internalization of relapse prevention measures and God's healing grace in my life, I have, for a number of years, felt ready to live a productive life in the free world once again, with positive goals in mind that are wholly incompatible with re-offending.

And yet in my journey to personal regeneration something was missing. There was a victim of my offense. Even though there had been no physical injuries to her, here was an innocent person who had undoubtedly suffered psychologically for a long time and deeply because of my criminal act. The missing component was that I had had no opportunity to meet with my victim, or communicate with her in any way to express to her my remorse for what I had done and seek her forgiveness, if she could give it. I was concerned that my victim still harbored a vengeful attitude toward me even with the passage of many years. My faith teaches me that vengeance is a two-edged sword with no handle. Those who try to use it become the injured and that is why only God can wield the sword of vengeance. Consequently, when I was able to meet with my victim, it was one of the most meaningful experiences of my life because I was finally able to have the opportunity to experience that missing component. The victim of my offense was empowered to respond to her own needs, as she saw them, to help heal the mental and emotional wounds that had been nagging at her for many years.

When the dialogue session began I was somewhat tense because no matter the amount of preparation that precedes such a meeting, there remain unknowns. But as my victim began speaking to open the dialogue session, I could sense that she had not come to grind an axe or to berate or demean me but, as I hoped she would, she came to do what she needed to do in order to bring as much healing and closure as possible to what occurred years ago. During the course of her statements to me she expressly forgave me (the man, not the act) and that compassionate, merciful act of her part surely freed her from aggravation and anger and the desire to strike back at me. When she told me that she forgave me, no longer hated or feared me, God touched my spirit at that instant, and I knew she was sincere and that she could go on with her life with a peace of mind and spirit she had not known for many years. You see, fear is a coward who is beaten when an injured human being can say, "I can" and "I will forgive." The capacity of a human being to forgive is unlimited. It is awesome when received and surely God-inspired to give. I don't know when my victim chose to forgive me but perhaps when she made that decision she shifted her eyes away from an image of me, the person who had hurt her, and set her eyes on the One who saved her, who saves us all with His redeeming grace. Forgiveness does not mean condoning or forgetting. It means giving up the feeling of being hostage to a traumatic event, of the right to be angry and the desire to strike back. Shortly after she forgave me I was reminded of Jesus, hanging on the cross, His words of invitation to the criminal hanging beside Him. With that act of forgiveness, Jesus provided an example to all mankind in every age.

Forgiveness is often a difficult principle to understand and apply in the present climate of harsh criminal justice policies. We as a society have a deep-rooted assumption that for every act there should be an equal reaction. Revenge and anger are powerful emotions. We can focus on simple solutions when we are angry. But until we can forgive we cannot move on. Faith and healing can inspire forgiveness, and forgiveness and reconciliation are ways to peace for victims of crimes and those who commit them.

The dialogue allowed me to look into the eyes of my victim and to express my sincere remorse to her for what I had done and to apologize in a way that she indicated was meaningful for her. She and I also discussed the ripple effect of crime, of my crime, and things we both had done over the years in reaching out to others who are affected by crime. I was able to share with her the effects of God's healing in my own life, how I have been able to confront and deal with the cognitive distortions that led me to offend. We both made certain commitments to undertake specific projects and work toward individual goals in the months and years ahead. The dialogue was a transforming experience, and I am certain that because of the experience both my victim and I have been able to restore, somewhat, our belief in the human family that is larger than both of us, yet incomplete without either of us. It was so important to me that my victim be able to feel a sense of being freed from the clutches of the criminal act itself, that she no longer hated me as a person.

The dominant theme of criminal justice today is generally punitive, very impersonal and state-centered. Both state and the federal governments have ratcheted up sentencing schemes to unprecedented levels. Contemporary criminal justice systems actually encourage offenders to deny responsibility for their crimes and empathy for their victims. Many prisoners would perhaps be unwilling to participate in the kind of victim-offender dialogue that was such a blessing to my victim and me. One reason for this reluctance is because many offenders feel that they cannot afford to admit their guilt. Overly harsh sentencing laws are part of the reason. Offenders sentenced to thirty, forty, sixty, ninety-nine years or life may very well spend five or ten years in the courts, challenging the validity of their convictions. Quite often offenders feel that they must maintain their innocence and, under some circumstances, a reviewing court may require a claim of "actual innocence" before agreeing to review a prisoner's claim. Of course, not all sentences meted out are disproportionate to the circumstances of crime committed, but some are. Regardless of the merits of arguments about appropriate sentencing of offenders, the practical result is that offenders are encouraged to deny personal responsibility for their crimes, particularly violent crimes. After so many years of imprisonment and dealing with criminal justice matters, it is clear to me that punitive criminal justice systems are unquestionably their own worst enemies, embittering many of those whom they confine, and serving neither the interests of victims, offenders, or their families.

There is another approach to crime and punishment, however, and it is known as "restorative justice." What happened in my case is an important component of that concept. Instead of focusing almost entirely upon punishment of offenders, as retributive systems do, restorative justice focuses on the harm resulting from crime, what needs to be done to repair that harm, and who is responsible for repairing that harm. The emphasis is on healing and the entire concept focuses on core values of personal responsibility, forgiveness and reconciliation. The restorative justice process recognizes what a quarter of a century in prison has shown me: that a punitive system does not recognize the "dignity" of *all* who are involved. Restorative justice encourages offenders to understand the harm they have caused to their victims and the ripple effect of the crimes. In the victim-offender dialogue process, for example, each person may come to the dialogue session with certain goals in mind. But each may leave with other, more specific or larger goals, transformed more by the experience itself than the participant could have imagined. In preparing for the dialogue session I had certain goals in mind. As I have previously mentioned, for many years I had wanted to speak with my victim in order to express my sincere remorse to her for what I had done to her, and to seek her forgiveness. In preparing for the dialogue I was also guided by certain goals of the program itself, as outlined by the mediator. Those goals included providing my victim with the opportunity to grieve unresolved trauma, to express to me the impact of the offense on her life, to ask questions about the offense that only I could answer, and to determine appropriate acts of restitution and constructive acts which would facilitate healing. Even with extensive preparation, one could not have predicted how my victim and I would interact when we actually met and when perhaps we would both be thrown back in time to when the crime occurred. But I had determined that whatever my victim's demeanor toward me, whatever her words to me, I would do what I could to help her bring what closure she could to the criminal act I had committed against her.

I was transformed by the actual dialogue session because the meeting exceeded my expectations in several ways. When I first saw my victim, after the passage of quite a number of years, I became somewhat tense and nervous. As the dialogue began, however, my victim expressed to me her thoughts and feelings in such a way that I knew that whatever the impact of my crime upon her, this courageous person had a measured heart for justice. She described to me the impact of the crime upon her life but she did it not with an angry or vengeful demeanor, but in a quiet and firm manner that imprinted on my mind the important information she was conveying to me. Over the years I had read some case studies of crimes in which victims write about the impact of crimes on their lives. But actually hearing about the impact of my crime upon my victim, first-hand, made an indelible impression upon me that I will never forget. As she continued with her statements to me she reached a point where she told me that she forgave me (the man, not the act) for what I had done to her. That was something that I prayed could happen, but did not know whether it would.

As our dialogue continued, I was able to express my remorse, and she accepted my remorse and apology in good faith. I sensed that she was empowered to express what she felt she needed to convey to me in order to facilitate her own healing. The uneasiness that characterized the early period of the dialogue session gave way to an atmosphere of an acceptance of what had happened in the past and that we both should move ahead and strive for the positive goals we had set for ourselves. We agreed on post-dialogue goals for each of us to accomplish. I was transformed by the experience because I had experienced genuine forgiveness from a person I had hurt and never got to know in an ordinary way.

Because my victim forgave me, I have the courage to live as a forgiven man. When engaging in criminal conduct I betrayed the values I had been raised to believe in. Values I had learned from my family, friends, and community–values which included the joy of clean living, the conviction that wealth is less than a good name, and respect for the dignity of all human beings. Having the courage to live as a forgiven man means that although I will not ever forget the criminal act I committed against my victim, I can go forward with my life with a renewed conscience and self-respect that will allow me to be a positive influence on others in my community, and with my own family. I can seek reconciliation with my own children and be at some degree of peace with myself because I have been forgiven by God, and now by my victim.

I am in my 50s now, and I guess I'm like an old barn. Barns, like people, reveal their characteristics as they season. I'm a bit droopy at the shoulders these days and have a tired back that sags in the middle. But like the old timbers of a weathered barn, I still persevere as long as I can hang by the nail that binds me to the cross of Christ, the one who redeemed me, the one who redeems in a way that lasts.

Later that same day, after the dialogue between my victim and me had concluded, I was back in my living quarters in the institution where I am confined. When giving thanks to God for the blessed experience of that day, I recalled something my mother said to me over twenty years ago while she and my father were visiting me in prison. She said she forgave me for the criminal act I had committed, and she commented that she fully expected me to come out of prison a renewed man, and live as the person I was raised to be. She encouraged me to renew and deepen my commitment to God. I promised her that I would, and it was a promise I was determined to keep. My parents passed away during the mid 1980s, but somehow I feel that they know that I have kept that promise.

The Texas Department of Criminal Justice is to be commended for the existence of its victim-offender dialogue program. My victim and I were blessed to have a compassionate mediator who conscientiously prepared us both for the actual dialogue meeting. The mediator's insights, when charting the largely unknown waters of the dialogue session, helped produce a result that surely helped contribute to the validation of the program. The entire dialogue session was filmed, and I understand is being used by the victim services division for training purposes and for facilitating the healing and recovery of crime victims. I also want to thank my victim, whose name I will not reveal here, whose courage in initiating the dialogue between us should give inspiration and hope to other victims about the possibilities of victim-offender dialogues.

The Texas victim services division does not, however, report the dialogue with my victim to the Texas parole board, or provide the parole board with a copy of the film of the dialogue. One would think most parole boards charged with gathering all available information pertaining to the parole readiness of an offender would be very interested in considering what occurred during the dialogue process. In all my years of experience with rehabilitative issues, I would be hard-pressed to think of a single event that had a more positive impact on my own regeneration that the fruitful dialogue that occurred between my victim and me. Approximately four months after the dialogue, I was again denied parole by the Texas parole board, for the fifteenth time, without being interviewed by any parole board decision-maker. In Texas, most all parole decisions are made by parole board members on the basis of undertaking a brief "paper review" of the offender's parole file. Certain categories of offenders may be singled out for blanket parole denials, based on considerations unrelated to parole readiness, no matter how parole ready any particular offenders in those targeted groups may be.

Victim-offender dialogues can produce extremely positive results to all parties involved. Without such a process victim healing is surely more difficult to achieve, and victims of crimes never have the opportunity to ask offenders questions about crimes that only the offender can answer. But if primarily retributive criminal justice systems are to be maintained, then the concept of "restorative justice" will end up playing a much smaller role than it should. More and more offenders are being sentenced to prison terms so harsh as to take away hope. Offenders are like anyone else. When they feel they have no hope they may easily be overcome by despair and develop an attitude of unwillingness to help themselves or anyone else. This is sad, because victim-offender dialogues can do for the participants what punitive justice can rarely accomplish, that is, help to heal victims and communities from effects of crime, and return offenders to society as truly law-abiding citizens who can make positive contributions to their communities. We need policy-makers and politicians who will create conditions that foster hope for all, that allow healing and closure to crimes to the maximum extent possible, rather than pandering to public misconceptions about criminal justice issues and riding the backs of offenders into office. I, for one, can only hope and pray that legislators and criminal justice officials will create conditions where "restorative justice" can become a part of the rehabilitation efforts of all offenders who are conscientious about reforming their lives and helping to repair the harm they have caused to their victims and communities, and indeed, to themselves and their own families.

I will conclude by saying that, in my case, the dialogue that occurred between my victim and me was something I had hoped would happen–that missing component in my own personal regeneration that, for me, could not have been fulfilled in any other way. I believe that the dramatic impact of victim-offender dialogues on an offender can become the motivation for the offender to begin to turn his life around. This is because of the transforming nature of the dialogue process, during which the offender may very well be able to begin to identify his own concerns about his criminal behavior, leading to his coming to terms with himself, able to articulate his new reasons for change, and reaching a conscious decision to turn his life around. There are thousands of crime victims who need the healing and some reasonable sense of closure that victim-offender dialogues can provide. There are thousands of offenders who truly desire to turn their lives around. Legislators and other policy makers should give these offenders hope, and encourage victims of these offenders to participate in the dialogue/reconciliation process that can produce the kind of positive results that occurred with me and the victim of my offense. What happened in my case is one of the great potentials of "restorative justice." With God's grace I will continue to live as a forgiven man, even though I remain incarcerated in an unforgiving criminal justice system.

Justice that Restores:
From Impersonal to Personal Justice

Daniel W. Van Ness

SUMMARY. Restorative justice is a movement within criminal justice that draws from a conception of justice as personal rather than impersonal. This article offers a definition of restorative justice and describes its hallmark programs: victim offender mediation, conferencing, circles, restitution, and community service. It explores the differences between restorative justice and contemporary criminal justice, including their relative strengths. Whereas criminal justice derives from an impersonal conception of justice, restorative justice draws from a personal understanding. Differences between the two views of justice are described, and a brief survey of history and cultures demonstrates that personal conceptions of justice have played, and continue to play, significant roles in shaping societies' responses to crime. *[Article copies available for a fee from The Haworth Document Delivery Service: 1-800-HAWORTH. E-mail address: <docdelivery@haworthpress.com> Website: <http://www.HaworthPress.com> © 2004 by The Haworth Press, Inc. All rights reserved.]*

Daniel W. Van Ness, JD, LLM, is Executive Director of the International Centre for Justice and Reconciliation, a criminal justice reform program of Prison Fellowship International.

Address correspondence to: Daniel W. Van Ness, PFI, PO Box 17434, Washington, DC 20041 (E-mail: dvanness@pfi.org).

[Haworth co-indexing entry note]: "Justice that Restores: From Impersonal to Personal Justice." Van Ness, Daniel W. Co-published simultaneously in *Journal of Religion & Spirituality in Social Work* (The Haworth Social Work Practice Press, an imprint of The Haworth Press, Inc.) Vol. 23, No. 1/2, 2004, pp. 93-109; and: *Criminal Justice: Retribution vs. Restoration* (ed: Eleanor Hannon Judah, and Rev. Michael Bryant) The Haworth Social Work Practice Press, an imprint of The Haworth Press, Inc., 2004, pp. 93-109. Single or multiple copies of this article are available for a fee from The Haworth Document Delivery Service [1-800-HAWORTH, 9:00 a.m. - 5:00 p.m. (EST). E-mail address: docdelivery@haworthpress.com].

http://www.haworthpress.com/web/JRSSW
© 2004 by The Haworth Press, Inc. All rights reserved.
Digital Object Identifier: 10.1300/J377v23n01_06

KEYWORDS. Restorative justice, victim offender mediation, conferencing, circles, restitution, community service

It was a hot day in Jericho. The temperature was hot, and so were emotions. Zacchaeus the tax collector was throwing his weight around again. First century tax collectors were collaborators with Rome, responsible for collecting money from their fellow citizens to pay for the empire's military reach. The Romans knew that the local population could fool a foreign tax collector, so they enlisted citizens of the occupied country to do the work. The inducement to the tax collectors was that they could keep whatever they collected above the amount Rome required. With the backing of Roman soldiers, these tax collectors became very wealthy.

Zacchaeus was the chief tax collector in the Jericho district. Nothing happened that he did not approve or profit from. The New Testament reports that tax collectors were hated (ranked with sinners and prostitutes), and Zacchaeus the ringleader would have been even more despised.

In times of tyranny, the oppressed make small gestures of defiance, and the citizens of Jericho did just that on this hot day. There was a special visitor coming through Jericho–Jesus of Nazareth. Some believed he was the Messiah, others that he was a great prophet. He seemed to have supernatural powers; he had brought dead people to life and healed sick people. He had fed large crowds and given a wedding party wine to drink out of jars of water. Some people felt that when he reached Jerusalem he would declare himself the Messiah and lead an uprising against Rome. The people of Jericho wanted to see him as he passed through.

Zacchaeus wanted to see him as well. The problem was that he was a short man who could not see over the assembled crowd. He pleaded, cajoled, and threatened, but the people would not let him through. He might be a big man on tax day, but today they would cut him down to size. Besides, why would he want to see Jesus? He was on Rome's side, and if Jesus were the long-expected King of the Jews, Zacchaeus would hardly want to welcome him. That is why emotions were hot. Zacchaeus wanted through; the people refused.

Giving up on getting through the crowd, Zacchaeus ran ahead and climbed a sycamore fig tree, common in Israel, and terrific for climbing with its strong low branches. He had picked his tree well, for Jesus' route came right past the tree. But when he reached the base of the tree,

Jesus stopped and looked up into the tree at Zacchaeus. The crowd grew still, waiting for the confrontation between this Holy Man and the corrupt traitor of Israel.

What did they expect Jesus to say? Undoubtedly, both they and Zacchaeus had similar ideas about the words that would come from Jesus' lips: words of denunciation, of condemnation. Just as John the Baptizer had denounced taxpayers' practices for years, Jesus would surely condemn Zacchaeus (Luke 19:1-10).

If Zacchaeus were tried under US law, rather than ancient Jewish law, it is reasonably clear what would happen. He would be charged with serious felonies and undoubtedly sentenced to a substantial prison sentence made longer under federal sentencing guidelines because of the amount of money earned through overcharging taxpayers. Newspapers would favorably editorialize that the sentence was necessary to send a message to other people in the public trust, and to the public as a whole, that laws must be obeyed.

If justice is seen as the impersonal application of objective standards to a person's behavior, then such a response could be defended as just. Laws must be upheld through punishment, if necessary. But there is an alternative conception of justice, one that we might call personal justice that does not end its work with vindication of the law. Instead, it also leads to an exploration of the material, personal, relational and spiritual dimensions of the harm caused by the wrongdoing. Accountability in this view has less to do with punishment and more to do with making amends (although it may be difficult and even painful).

This article begins with a short introduction to restorative justice and its hallmark programs, it draws distinctions between restorative justice and contemporary criminal justice, and it reviews the ways that personal conceptions of justice are interwoven with impersonal conceptions in diverse cultures and in legal history.

INTRODUCTION TO RESTORATIVE JUSTICE

Restorative justice is a movement within the criminal justice system that focuses more attention on the harm to victims and communities and less on the fact of lawbreaking (Zehr, 1990). A number of definitions of restorative justice have been proposed, some focusing on its distinctive decision-making processes and others on its reparative outcomes. A definition that includes all those is the following:

Restorative justice is a systematic response to wrongdoing that emphasizes healing the wounds of victims, offenders, and communities caused or revealed by crime. Practices and programs reflecting restorative purposes will respond to crime by: (1) identifying and taking steps to repair harm, (2) involving all stakeholders, and (3) transforming the traditional relationship between communities and their governments in responding to crime. (Van Ness & Crocker, 2003)

Three programs have become closely identified with restorative justice processes: victim offender mediation, conferencing, and circles. Two other programs have been acknowledged as providing potentially restorative outcomes: restitution and community service. Looking at each of these in turn will help expand on the definition offered above.

Victim Offender Mediation

The first contemporary restorative process was victim offender mediation. In its prototypical form, this programme brings together victims and their offenders, using a trained facilitator to coordinate and facilitate the meeting. In the course of the meeting, the victims describe their experiences with the crime and the effect it has had on them. The offenders explain what they did and why, answering questions the victim may have. When both victim and offender have had their say, the facilitator will help them consider ways to make things right. Typically, the facilitator will have met with each party prior to their meeting to prepare them (see Figure 1), although in some European countries, mediation does not necessarily involve a direct meeting between the two parties. Instead, the facilitator conducts shuttle negotiation with each party until an agreement on restitution is reached (Umbreit, 2001).

Victim offender mediation can take place at any time during the criminal justice process, or outside the system altogether. Like the other restorative processes, it will occur after guilt is no longer an issue either because there has been a conviction or because the defendant admits responsibility. It can take place before sentencing or after. It may have an effect on the sentence or it may have no effect, depending on the laws or regulations in place.

Conferencing

Conferencing developed in New Zealand as an alternative to Youth Courts. It was adapted from traditional processes of the Maori people,

FIGURE 1. Victim Offender Mediation

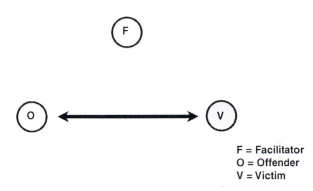

F = Facilitator
O = Offender
V = Victim

the indigenous population there. Conferencing has been further adapted in other countries, and there are now several versions of conferencing (New Zealand Maori Council & Hull, 1999).

Conferencing differs from mediation in that it involves more parties in the process. Not only are the primary victim and offender included, so are secondary victims (such as family members or friends of the victim) as well as supporters of the offender (such as family members and friends). These people are involved because they have also been affected in some way by the offence, and because they care about one of the primary participants. They may also participate in carrying out the final agreement. In addition, representatives of the criminal justice system may participate (see Figure 2) (McCold, 1999).

The conference has a facilitator who arranges for the meeting and makes sure that everyone present is able to participate fully. The facilitator does not play a role in the substantive discussions. Some forms of conferencing are "scripted," which means that the facilitator follows a prescribed pattern in guiding discussion by the participants (O'Connell, Wachtel, & Wachtel, 1999). Conferencing is used in multiple stages of the criminal justice process, but it has typically been used earlier than victim offender mediation. In fact, conferencing is used by police as an alternative to arrest and referral to the formal criminal justice process (Young & Hoyle, 2003). This has led to unique linkages between restorative justice and the formal justice system.

Circles

Circles are similar to conferencing in that they expand participation beyond the primary victim and offender: Their families and supporters

FIGURE 2. Conferencing

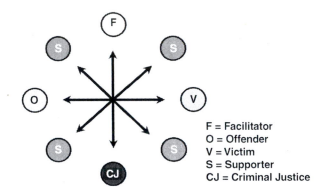

F = Facilitator
O = Offender
V = Victim
S = Supporter
CJ = Criminal Justice

may attend, as well as criminal justice personnel. But in addition, any member of the community who has an interest in the case may come and participate, making circles the most inclusive process of the three (see Figure 3).

Circles draw from First Nations practices in Canada, and they retain some of that flavor (Green, 1998). All the participants sit in a circle. Typically, the offender begins with an explanation of what happened, and then everyone around the circle is given the opportunity to talk. The discussion moves from person to person, clockwise, around the circle. Anyone may say what he or she wishes. Conversation continues until everything that needs to be said has been said, and they come to resolution. The facilitator is known as the Keeper of the circle. This person's role, like that of the facilitator in the other two processes, is to ensure that the process is protected. There is a talking piece as well, which may be a feather or some other object that has meaning to members of the circle. The talking piece is passed around the circle, and only the person holding it is permitted to speak (Pranis, 1997).

Circles are used at various stages of the justice process. They are also used independently of criminal justice to address community or group problems that may not have risen to the level of criminal activity or which are not likely to lead to criminal charges. Sometimes called healing circles or community circles, these may not include all the parties: Healing circles, for example, may involve only the victim and the victim's supporters or the offender and the offender's supporters (Stuart, 1996).

FIGURE 3. Circles

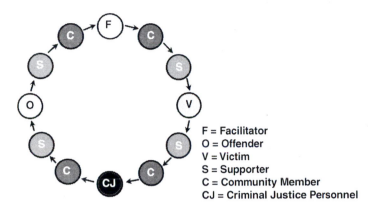

F = Facilitator
O = Offender
V = Victim
S = Supporter
C = Community Member
CJ = Criminal Justice Personnel

Those three programmes might be seen as examples of encounter programs. They make it possible for victims, offenders and other stakeholders to actually meet each other to discuss what took place, the injustice that was involved, the harm that resulted, and how to make amends. How can an offender make amends? There are several ways in which this often occurs. One is through an apology, a sincere admission of what the offender has done, and an expression of regret for having done that. Apologies are a common result of the encounter programs mentioned above (Cavanagh, 1998). However, there are two additional forms of amends that are more tangible in nature.

Restitution

One is restitution, where the offender pays back the victim for the harm caused. Restitution can be made through financial payments, by return or replacement of property, or by performing direct services for the victim, or in any way that the parties agree (Harland, 1982). Restitution can be imposed on an unwilling offender at the conclusion of court proceedings, but in such a situation, the "restorative" character of restitution will be limited to the reparation the victim receives, which should not be discounted. Under those circumstances the opportunities for explanation, expression of feelings, apology, and other relational interactions are absent. Restitution will have a more restorative effect when it results from a restorative process.

Community Service

This is also true of community service, the second common way of making amends. Community service involves the offender providing free services to a charitable or governmental agency. Community service can be imposed, and the practice in many countries has been that the service required has little relationship to the offence or the harm it caused. When used that way, it is little more than a retributive sanction with minimal if any restorative impact. However, even imposed community service can have some restorative effect if (1) the service follows a restorative process between the victim and offender, (2) community members are involved in determining the kind of service that will be meaningful to the community and the offender, (3) community members and the offender perform the service side by side, (4) there is public acknowledgement of the offender's contribution, (5) there are opportunities for reflection so that the service is seen as giving to the community, and (6) the offender has an opportunity to develop competencies (Pranis, Bazemore, Umbreit, & Lipkin, 1998). Finally, it is important that the community service not be selected because it is degrading or humiliating. When that does happen, community service becomes simply another form of punishment. As with restitution, the more that community service comes out of restorative processes, the more restorative it will be as an outcome.

RESTORATIVE JUSTICE AND CONTEMPORARY CRIMINAL JUSTICE

The foundation of contemporary criminal justice is that crime is viewed as lawbreaking, which means that justice requires us to uphold the authority of the government by punishing the offender. This means that the main focuses of criminal justice are on retribution (when it looks back to the lawbreaking), on deterrence and incapacitation (when it looks toward a future with less crime), and on the offender as the lawbreaker.

Restorative justice pioneer Howard Zehr (2002) has suggested that the central questions in a criminal proceeding are: "What laws have been broken?" "Who did it?" and "What do they deserve?" (p. 21). Answers to the first two questions are given when the accused defendant pleads guilty or is found guilty following a full-fledged criminal trial. Judges answer the final question based on the sentencing policies of the jurisdiction. Generally, those policies revolve around deterrence, incapacitation, rehabilitation, and retribution. Restorative justice begins at a different point. The reason certain acts are criminalized is to prevent harm to the common good. Assuming that laws are just, a person who commits a crime violates the common good, causes or threatens to cause harm.

When crimes do occur, a restorative response focuses on the harm to victims, to communities, and even to those who commit the crimes. Justice is understood as repairing those harms, and in particular requiring that the offender assume primary responsibility in making amends. The focus of restorative justice is on reparation to the victim (when it looks back at the harm caused by the offence), on reintegration of the victim and offender (when it looks forward to a future with less crime), and on the victim as the person who was most directly harmed by the offence.

It is not surprising that a restorative response asks different questions about what justice requires in the aftermath of a crime: Zehr proposes the following three as alternatives to those posed by traditional criminal justice: "Who has been hurt?" "What are their needs?" and "Whose obligations are these?" (Zehr, 1990, p. 21). The first question moves beyond considering whether lawbreaking has been proved to examining the harm that resulted. The second question changes the focus from a preoccupation with the accused defendant to concern for the victimized individuals and communities; the victim should be central under this way of thinking about crime. The third question emphasizes the need for accountability and reparation by the offender, and perhaps by the community as well. A just response is one that makes things right.

Each approach claims certain strengths. The criminal justice system emerged over centuries of development, and it has important features that should not be given up lightly. One of these is the recognition that there should be safeguards provided to people accused of crimes. These rights are not always honored, and critics may point to absurd consequences when these are taken to extremes. But one would want to think carefully before giving them up.

Criminal justice is also good at exhibiting social condemnation of criminal acts. Its power of denunciation is considerable. Criminal justice provides an alternative to personal or collective vengeance, which could lead to cycles of vengeance and violence. Furthermore, it offers a more efficient process by having professional police, public prosecutors, governmental prison systems and so on rather than expecting individual victims to prosecute.

Finally, at its best criminal justice aspires to overall fairness–working toward consistency of punishment for similar crimes, for example. This is an elusive goal, but it is one that criminal justice takes seriously (at least in theory).

The strengths of restorative justice begin with its more holistic view of crime, recognizing the harm that results, and not the lawbreaking alone. It measures success not by the amount of punishment imposed, but by the amount of damage that has been repaired. Its focus on harm means that it should take the needs of victims seriously (although restorative programmes do not always do so). It recognizes that there is a need for community participation in society's response to crime, rather than leaving this to the government alone. And it offers considerably more flexibility in how particular cases are handled.

IMPERSONAL AND PERSONAL CONCEPTIONS OF JUSTICE

Criminologist Herbert Packer (1968) has suggested that there are essentially two models of criminal justice. The crime control model includes all the strategies that place the highest value on suppression of criminal conduct. Under the due process model, he placed any policies, programs, laws, and so forth whose purpose is to restrain government from abusing its power.

John Griffiths (1970) responded that rather than providing two models, Packer had really offered only one, which Griffiths called the battle model. Both Packer's proposed models viewed criminal justice as a struggle between two forces with irreconcilable interests: the government and the person suspected of being a criminal. Griffiths argued that when viewed this way, Packer's models were not dichotomies at all, but simply variations on the single theme of battle. To demonstrate the significance of looking for a true alternative to that single theme, he proposed: the family model of criminal justice. Where Packer assumed disharmony, Griffiths proposed a personal conception of justice, one that assumes "reconcilable–even mutually supportive–interests, a state of love" (p. 371). Crime and punishment would be treated significantly differently than under a model which views the criminal as a deviant and outlaw. It is not clear whether Griffiths was seriously proposing a new model, or simply demonstrating the limitations of Packer's. But his suggestion that conflict be seen as reconcilable rather than as fatal is central to restorative justice theory.

Criminal justice derives from an impersonal and formal conception of justice: Government defends official norms by identifying the person who has violated those norms, determining his or her guilt, and then imposing a sanction on the guilty. Traditionally, sanctioning is seen as performing one or more of four purposes. It may deter the offender and/or others who might have become offenders because of the degree and kind of punishment imposed. It may incapacitate offenders by physically preventing them from being able to commit another offence through prison, curfews, and so forth. It might rehabilitate by changing the offender so that he or she becomes law abiding. Finally, it may simply be retribution, punishment because it is deserved and not because it serves a utilitarian purpose. All of these purposes are believed to help suppress criminal behavior, and would be included in Packer's crime control model.

Because of government's power, as well as the potential severity of the sanctions, defendants in criminal procedures are afforded certain rights and protections. These rights, to be honored even when the accused person is guilty, include due process rights, which concern how the person is to be treated by the police, courts and sanctioning authorities, and rights stemming from basic human dignity, which concern issues such as cruel and inhuman treatment or punishment. These examples would be included in Packer's due process model.

The alternative to impersonal justice is personal and informal justice. This is what characterizes justice in a family, which was Griffiths' model. It also occurs when one friend has wronged another, or if a person with certain values harms even a stranger. The wrongdoing is followed by confession, apology, an attempt to make amends if necessary, perhaps forgiveness, and the matter is resolved. This conception of justice can be referred to as personal in two ways. First, it is carried out by the people in the conflict themselves, sometimes with the help of others as facilitators. Decisions are made jointly by the victim, the offender and other interested parties in a process of dialogue and negotiation. Justice is done by the parties, not to them. Second, justice is personal because its objectives are personal. The goal of personal justice is to restore the parties to healthy, productive relationships within their communities. This requires clarification of the norms and values of the parties and of the community around them, but it discovers those norms and values in the course of conversation and not merely by consulting statute books.

Personal justice is not indifferent to objective standards of right and wrong, but it does not stop with that consideration. It goes beyond that to reflect on the harm caused or revealed by the wrongdoing, and seeks ways to restore community wholeness. The category of persons harmed certainly includes the victim, but can also include secondary victims and sometimes even the community itself, and because their interests are at stake, they are given a voice in the process.

PERSONAL JUSTICE IN HISTORY

From the times of the ancient legal codes of the Middle East to the medieval kingdoms of Europe and England, those administering justice were preoccupied with preserving community harmony. They took crime seriously because it threatened the common welfare, but they did so by ensuring that the victim received satisfaction. It was not until European and English rulers began centralizing power and consolidating small kingdoms into large that crime came to be viewed as an offense against the government, rather than against the victim (Berman, 1983).

The Classical Greeks recognized the importance of a personal understanding of justice. Aristotle argued that law alone is insufficient in pursuing justice. Since law is universal, abstract, and impersonal, but disputes are particular, concrete, and personal, he reasoned that there would be occasions when law would not be able to achieve justice, and he provided for equity.

> Equity bids us be merciful to the weakness of human nature; to think less about the laws than about the man who framed them, and less about what he said than about what he meant; not to consider the actions of the accused so much as his intentions, nor this or that detail so much as the whole story; to ask not what a man is now but what he has always or usually been. It bids us remember benefits rather than injuries, and benefits received rather than benefits conferred; to be patient when we are wronged; to settle a dispute by negotiation and not by force; to prefer arbitration to litigation—for an arbitrator goes by the equity of a case, a judge by the strict law, and arbitration was invented with the express purpose of securing full power for equity. (Aristotle, Book I, Sec. 13, Lines 11-23)

It was important for offenders and their families to make amends to the victims and their families. They sought peace through negotiation and reconciliation rather than through imposed public order. They understood crime to be a community event involving victims, offenders, and their kin. Their response was to secure community peace by requiring offenders to make amends (Hoebel, 1973). They sought reparation for victims–not simply to insure that victims received restitution, but also as part of a process of restoring community peace.

This is evident even in the terminology employed. The ancient Hebrew word *shalom* means peace, harmony, completeness, fulfillment, and wholeness. Shalom describes a community in which everyone is in right relationship with other individuals, the community as a whole, and God (Carr, 1980). This was understood to be a community's ideal condition, an ideal seldom reached for many reasons, one of which was crime. Crime destroys right relationships and sows distrust and fear within a community. So, the ancient Hebrew justice portrayed in the scriptures aimed to restore those broken relationships to wholeness. Restitution was considered essential, not only for what it would do for the victim but also for the community as a whole. The Hebrew word for "restitution" is *shillum* and comes from the same root as shalom (Carr, 1980). In other words, restitution was understood to be a way of reconciling the parties and reestablishing community peace, shalom.

Furthermore, the law was to be vindicated. The word for this is *shillem,* which comes from the same root word as shalom and shillum. Shillem means "retribution" or "recompense" in the sense of satisfaction, or vindication (Carr, 1980). So, doing justice would restore peace and harmony by repaying the victim and upholding community values expressed in the law.

This recognition of a personal dimension to justice continued in Anglo-American legal history. In England, the Courts of Equity emerged as a response to the injustices of an increasingly inflexible common law. Litigants who complained of an unjust result because of technicalities or arcane formalities could apply to the King's Chancellor for relief, extended in the name of the King. Over time, the requests became so frequent, and the principles of relief so well established, that professional judges were appointed to hear cases, precedent began to accumulate and a new, formal, substantive law emerged (Baker, 1990).

There are other examples of the recognition of personal justice in our legal history. In American colonial times, Magistrate's Courts were effectively emancipated from the common law and from lawyers, both viewed by many as confusing and perverting justice (Baker, 1990). The rehabilitation model of criminal sentencing arose in the eighteenth century as a means of personalizing and individualizing justice. Inmates were placed in isolation and provided the assistance their keepers believed that each one needed. This led ultimately to the indeterminate sentence, which guaranteed that the prisoners would be treated until their rehabilitation was completed (Morris & Rothman, 1995). The jury began in England as a method of including relational and informal strengths within the emerging criminal justice system and it remains, in a highly diluted form, the most personal element of a system increasingly characterized by impersonal and formal elements such as "three strikes" laws and other mandatory sentencing provisions (Van Ness, 1994).

The personal conception of justice continues in non-Western cultures. Many pre-colonial African societies were compensatory and reconciliatory in nature, and as contemporary nations move away from their colonial heritage, some are recovering those features (Tutu, 1999).

The Japanese formal legal system is supplemented by a flourishing and organic informal system that fits the Japanese character and culture more effectively than do the laws. Going to law is a last resort for the Japanese, in part because of the Japanese character, but also because the laws and court systems are foreign to their culture. They would much rather deal with crime through apology and restitution, followed by changed behavior. An apology of a person who persists in wrongdoing is not well received because it is not believed. Such a person will have their case handled in the formal criminal justice system (Wagatsuma & Rosett, 1986).

While this has been a brief survey, intended to be suggestive rather than exhaustive, it is clear that personal conceptions of justice have played a significant role within Anglo-American legal traditions, in penology, and in other cultures. It demonstrates that restorative justice is not unique as an attempt to inject a personal justice perspective to what might otherwise be a highly impersonal justice system.

CONCLUSION

One of the schools of thought within the restorative justice movement is known as relational justice (Burnside & Baker, 1994). The name is an excellent one, because it emphasizes that at the heart of restorative justice is a focus on the persons involved in crime, and the relationships they brought into that experience and that were created by the experience. This article has suggested that restorative justice is just from the perspective of a personal understanding of justice. From the perspective of impersonal justice, it has limitations such as the low value given to proportionality and other safeguards (Ashworth, 1993).

With well-crafted guidelines or standards, however, restorative justice can direct attention past lawbreaking to forms of accountability that help repair crime (UN, 2002). It has the potential of responding to crime today as Jesus did with Zacchaeus.

There are four lines of dialogue in the account of Zacchaeus' meeting with Jesus. The first was spoken by Jesus as he came to the sycamore tree and noticed Zacchaeus sitting there. "Come down from the tree, Zacchaeus. I want to go to your house for dinner today." By having Zacchaeus come down to the ground, Jesus brought him together with his community, his victims. He created a meeting place right there in the shade of the sycamore tree.

Inviting himself to Zacchaeus' house was consistent with how Jesus had interacted with tax collectors before. One of his followers, Matthew, was a tax collector when he left his job to follow Jesus. One of the first things Matthew did was organize a dinner and invite his former colleagues to meet Jesus. But under these circumstances, a public invitation of this sort was guaranteed to be controversial. The people in the crowd began to murmur and complain. "He has gone to be the guest of a sinner!" they said. We can imagine their disappointment in Jesus. It looked as though he was siding with Zacchaeus. How is it possible? This second line of dialogue probably summarizes many things that the crowd said. In this single line, we hear the stories of many victims. Jesus' provocative opening line had given a voice to the people Zacchaeus had wronged for so many years.

The third line of dialogue belongs to Zacchaeus, and makes clear that the victim stories have affected him. "If I have stolen anything from anyone, I will pay back four times what I took. And after that, I will give half my goods to the poor in Jericho." Zacchaeus wants to make things right. To do this he returns to the Hebrew law with its provisions for restitution as a way of restoring community peace. Multiple amounts of restitution was a common provision, and Zacchaeus here accepts his responsibility to make right the harm he has caused. In fact, he goes beyond the requirements of the law and offers to give half his goods to the poor.

The final line belongs to Jesus: "Salvation has come to Zacchaeus' house, for he too is a son of Abraham." Everyone there counted himself or herself a son or daughter of Abraham. It is part of what gave them identity as a people. Through his behavior, Zacchaeus had placed himself outside this community, this extended family. Now after confession and in light of his efforts to make amends, Zacchaeus had found re-entry into that community. He had rejoined the family.

REFERENCES

Ashworth, A. (1993). Some doubts about restorative justice. *Criminal Law Forum, 4(2)*, 277-299.

Aristotle. (1924). Rhetorica. In W. D. Ross (Ed.), *The Works of Aristotle* (W. R. Roberts, Trans.). Oxford, England: Oxford University Press.

Baker, J. H. (1990). *An introduction to English legal history, 3rd edition.* London, England: Butterworths.

Berman, H. (1983). *Law and revolution: The formation of the Western legal tradition.* Cambridge, MA: Harvard University Press.

Burnside, J. & Baker, N. (Eds.) (1994). *Relational justice: Repairing the breach.* Winchester, England: Waterside Press.

Carr, G. L. (1980). Shalom. In R. L. Harris, G. R. Archer, Jr., & B. K. Waltke (Eds.), *Theological wordbook of the Old Testament* (p. 931). Chicago, IL: Moody Press.

Cavanagh, T. (1998). Adopting new values for the courts: What is restorative justice? *The Court Manager, 13(2/3)*, 24-27. Williamsburg, VA: National Association for Court Management.

Green, R. G. (1998). *Justice in aboriginal communities: Sentencing alternatives.* Saskatoon, Saskatchewan: Purich.

Griffiths, J. (1970). Ideology in criminal procedure or a third 'model' of the criminal process. *Yale Law Review, 79(3)*, 359-417.

Harland, A. T. (1982). Monetary remedies for the victims of crime: Assessing the role of the criminal courts. *UCLA Law Review, 30(1)*, 52-128.

Hoebel, A. E. (1973). *The law of primitive man: A study in comparative legal dynamics.* New York, NY: Atheneum.

McCold, P. (1999). *Restorative justice practice: The state of the field 1999.* A paper presented for the Building Strong Partnerships for Restorative Practices conference, Burlington, VT.

Morris, N. & Rothman, D. (1995). *The Oxford history of the prison: The practice of punishment in Western society.* New York, NY: Oxford University Press.

New Zealand Maori Council & Hull, D. D. (1999). Restorative justice: A Maori perspective. In Consedine, J. & Bowen, H. (Eds.), *Restorative justice: Contemporary themes and practice* (pp. 25-35). Lyttelton, NZ: Ploughshares.

O'Connell, T., Wachtel B., & Wachtel, T. (1999). *Conferencing handbook: The new REAL Justice training manual.* Pipersville, PA: The Piper's Press.

Packer, H. L. (1968). *The limits of the criminal sanction.* Stanford, CA: Stanford University Press.

Pranis, K. (1997). *Restoring community: The process of circle sentencing.* A paper presented for the Justice Without Violence: Views from Peacemaking Criminology and Restorative Justice conference.

Pranis, K., Bazemore, G., Umbreit M. S., & Lipkin R. (1998). *Guide for implementing the balanced and restorative justice model.* Washington, DC: Office of Juvenile Justice and Delinquency Prevention.

Stuart, B. (1996). Circle sentencing: Turning swords into ploughshares. In B. Galaway & J. Hudson (Eds.), *Restorative justice: International perspectives* (pp. 193-208). Monsey, NY: Criminal Justice Press.

Tutu, D. (1999). *No future without forgiveness*. New York, NY: Doubleday.

Umbreit, M. S. (2001). *The handbook of victim offender mediation: An essential guide to practice and research*. San Francisco, CA: Jossey-Bass.

United Nations. Economic and Social Council. Substantive Session 2002. (1-26 July 2002). *2002/12: Basic Principles on the Use of Restorative Justice Programmes in Criminal Matters*.

Van Ness, D. W. (1994). Preserving a community voice: The case for half-and-half juries in racially-charged criminal cases. *John Marshall Law Review, 28(1)*, 1-56.

Van Ness, D. W. & Crocker, C. E. (2003). Restorative justice: Definition, principles, values, and goals. *Restorative Justice Online*. Retrieved February 1, 2003, from the World Wide Web: http://www.restorativejustice.org/rj3/RJ_City/rjcity_defetc.htm

Wagatsuma, H. & Rosett, A. (1986). The implications of apology: Law and culture in Japan and the United States. *Law and Society Review, 20*, 461-98.

Young, R. & Hoyle, C. (2003). New, improved police-led restorative justice? In von Hirsch, A., Roberts, J., Bottoms, A. E., Roach, K., & Schiff, M. (Eds.), *Restorative justice & criminal justice: Competing or reconcilable paradigms?* (pp. 273-291). Oxford, England: Hart Publishing.

Zehr, H. (1990). *Changing lenses: A new focus for crime and justice*. Scottdale, PA: Herald Press.

Zehr, H. (2002). *The little book of restorative justice*. Intercourse, PA: Good Books.

Emerging Issues:
The Faith Communities
and the Criminal Justice System

Daniel J. Misleh
Evelyn U. Hanneman

SUMMARY. Restorative Justice is coming into focus for many faith communities as an important shift in response to crime. This paper examines the history of our response to crime and describes the response of a number of faith communities. Extended treatment is given to the November 2000 statement by the United States Catholic Bishops, *Re-*

Daniel J. Misleh, MTS, is Director of Diocesan Relations, Department of Social Development and World Peace, United States Conference of Catholic Bishops, Washington, DC. Mr. Misleh was a policy advisor on criminal justice issues in the Office of Domestic Social Development within the department and the primary staff person overseeing the bishops' statement *Responsibility, Rehabilitation and Restoration: A Catholic Perspective on Crime and Criminal Justice.* Address correspondence to: 3211 4th Street, NE, Washington, DC 20017 (E-mail: dmisleh@usccb.org).

Evelyn U. Hanneman, MS, is Restorative Justice Project Director, Baptist Peace Fellowship of North America and editor of *Kaleidoscope of Justice: Highlighting Restorative Juvenile Justice,* the quarterly newsletter of the Balanced and Restorative Justice Project. She has worked for 8 years to bring restorative justice to the criminal justice system in Maine while serving as Director of the Criminal Justice Program for the Maine Council of Churches. Address correspondence to: Baptist Peace Fellowship, 4800 Wedgewood Drive, Charlotte, NC 28210 (E-mail: evelyn@bpfna.org).

[Haworth co-indexing entry note]: "Emerging Issues: The Faith Communities and the Criminal Justice System." Misleh, Daniel J., and Evelyn U. Hanneman. Co-published simultaneously in *Journal of Religion & Spirituality in Social Work* (The Haworth Social Work Practice Press, an imprint of The Haworth Press, Inc.) Vol. 23, No. 1/2, 2004, pp. 111-131; and: *Criminal Justice: Retribution vs. Restoration* (ed: Eleanor Hannon Judah, and Rev. Michael Bryant) The Haworth Social Work Practice Press, an imprint of The Haworth Press, Inc., 2004, pp. 111-131. Single or multiple copies of this article are available for a fee from The Haworth Document Delivery Service [1-800-HAWORTH, 9:00 a.m. - 5:00 p.m. (EST). E-mail address: docdelivery@ haworthpress.com].

http://www.haworthpress.com/web/JRSSW
Digital Object Identifier: 10.1300/J377v23n01_07

sponsibility, Rehabilitation and Restoration: A Catholic Perspective on Crime and Criminal Justice. Their approach to crime and criminal justice is reviewed, including a special emphasis on the Catholic Church's teaching on the option for the poor and includes policy recommendations for church and society. Examples of activity at the local, state and national levels are given. The paper documents some effects of the bishops' statement on community and legislative activity at the local, state and national levels. *[Article copies available for a fee from The Haworth Document Delivery Service: 1-800-HAWORTH. E-mail address: <docdelivery@haworthpress.com> Website: <http://www.HaworthPress.com> © 2004 by The Haworth Press, Inc. All rights reserved.]*

KEYWORDS. Christian churches, faith communities, charitable choice, United States Catholic Bishops

INTRODUCTION

In this paper we show how the religious community, particularly the Christian community in the United States, is involved in criminal justice issues. From our biblical roots to today, the church has helped to shape approaches to crime, punishment, rehabilitation, and restoration of both offenders and victims. This history is no doubt checkered, but the core values of community, active participation, care for neighbors, compassion, justice, peace, and love eventually rise to the top when confronted with some of the toughest issues in this arena.

After a brief historical overview, concrete examples are given of some Christian denominations' responses to the call for restorative approaches to crime for the offender, the victim, and the community, and away from today's punitive retributive treatment of offenders with its lack of attention to victims and community. The recent document by the Catholic Bishops will be highlighted with its in-depth look at the criminal justice system in the U.S. and the need for a restorative response. In addition, the Catholic Church has provided funding for a number of grassroots programs based on restorative justice; an overview of several of these programs is then given.

Historical Overview

Scripture and religious tradition hold up the promise of *shalom*, living together in a community built on right relationships, to a world that all too often places confidence in individuality and detachment. Such a community could be said to be a place of peace based on justice. Peace in this context is not the absence of war or conflict but the presence of justice in all those dimensions that make for a well-lived life in community.

> The state of shalom is the state of flourishing in all dimensions of one's existence: in one's relation to God, in one's relations to one's fellow human beings, in one's relation to nature, and in one's relation to oneself. (Wolterstorff, 1999, p. 113)

This lack of shalom is very evident in the criminal justice system found in most of the Western world. The actual victim is removed from the process and the state becomes the victim. The focus is on the offender and how to punish him/her for the misdeeds. Nowhere is there concern to repair the harm caused by the crime done to the actual people involved; therefore, the process does not allow for healing to take place and a sense of shalom, as found in a healthy community, to be re-established or, perhaps, secured for the first time. Thus, one could state that in our criminal justice system true justice is seldom found.

This was not always the case. Crime was viewed in as harm done to individuals and the harmony of the community. The focus was on repairing this harm, which threatened the harmony of the community, through use of restitution. The victim might also demand vindication, that is, an acknowledgment that the wrong had been done to him/her. Both of these required the offender to accept responsibility for his/her actions, and to act to put things right, repairing the harm. Following a time of negotiations, a public declaration of fault would be given and payment of restitution made to the victim.

Most disputes were settled by the victim, or the victim's family, outside the courts within the context of the community. Justice was seen as a mediation and negotiation process with church and community leaders playing a major role. Agreements for restitution would be officially registered (Zehr, 1990).

Change came as the European and English rulers sought to consolidate power and wealth into their own hands and remove it from both the church and local authorities. Thus new laws decreed that crimes were to be dealt with in the King's Court instead of through the local communities, with fines paid to the king, sometimes in place of restitution paid to the victim. Through this, the Western world began to move from understanding crimes as being against individuals, to be dealt with in the context of community, to crimes being against the State with the court deciding the outcome and fines being paid to the State (Van Ness & Strong, 1997).

Over the past twenty years, the faith community has been reasserting its call for shalom through a renewed focus on the harm done by crime to all those involved, in the paradigm called restorative justice (Zehr, 1990). While there is movement in this direction from a number of other quarters, including community policing and the courts in what some call community justice, the faith community may hold the best hope for inspiring a justice system based on the wholeness encompassed in the term shalom. This paradigm seeks to put things right through holding offenders accountable to their victims in the context of community. Responsibility, reparation, and restitution are all part of restorative justice. The involvement of the community in all aspects is vitally important; otherwise restorative justice is simply one more program run by the system.

With the passage of the "charitable choice" provisions of the Personal Responsibility and Work Opportunity Reconciliation Act of 1996 (P.L. 104-93), there are new opportunities for religious organizations to work for change in the way the criminal justice system handles both offenders and victims. Because of the history of religious organizations' involvement and even in the founding of the criminal justice system itself and the unique role that they play in counseling both victims and offenders, it is hoped that many will embrace this new openness on the part of the government. The ability of religious organizations to compete for federal funds for programs targeted for victims, offenders, former offenders, and their families should be seen as an incentive to renew and re-engage their efforts in these areas.

CHURCH INVOLVEMENT IN RESTORATIVE JUSTICE

Most observers credit the Mennonite Church in Canada with the initial foray in recent years into restorative justice. Two Mennonites who were involved with the probation department in Kitchner, Ontario, proposed the daring notion of having two young offenders meet their victims (whose properties they had vandalized) to apologize and negotiate appropriate restitution. When the judge agreed, the first known victim offender mediations took place. Out of this developed the Victim Offender Reconciliation Program (VORP), which today has over 100 programs still primarily based in local churches throughout the U.S. and Canada. In a study of VORPs, over 80 percent of participating victims and offenders stated that they felt justice had been done, with a common theme being that things "had been made right" (Zehr, 1990).

Many faith communities have passed resolutions on restorative justice as a biblically based response needed to do justice today. In their materials, several focus on Micah 6:8, "You have been told, O man [sic], what is good, and what the Lord requires of you: only to do right and to love goodness, and to walk humbly with your God." Some offer materials for study and discussion; others include conferences and Websites to highlight restorative justice information.

Mennonite

The Mennonite Central Committee's U.S. Office on Crime and Justice provides information and resources on ministry to victims and offenders, victim offender reconciliation/conferencing, restorative justice, the death penalty and other related issues. It also coordinates presentations, workshops, and written material on restorative justice principles and their application, provides consultation and information to individuals and groups involved in victim offender reconciliation/conferencing programs (VORPs); and develops educational and training materials on various crime and justice issues.

Presbyterian

The Presbyterian Church USA (PCUSA) has focused on criminal justice issues for decades. Each February, PCUSA sponsors a Criminal Justice Sunday. For the past three years, the focus of this special Sunday has been on restorative justice. Their resources include videos, resources for those doing prison ministry, and a new justice curriculum, *Justice or "Just Desserts?": An Adult Study of the Restorative Justice Approach.* Covering four ninety-minute sessions, the course takes participants through a survey of the present criminal justice system, a discussion of what justice means, an explanation of restorative justice theory and its application to a case study, and a brainstorming session examining what a congregation can do within the church and the larger community.

United Methodist

The United Methodist Church (UMC) approved a resolution on restorative justice at their May 2000 General Conference. It states, in part:

> In the love of Christ, who came to save those who are lost and vulnerable, we urge the creation of a genuinely new system for the care and restoration of victims, offenders, criminal justice officials, and the community as a whole. Restorative Justice grows out of biblical authority, which emphasizes a right relationship with God, self and community. When such relationships are violated or broken through crime, opportunities are created to make things right . . . Through God's transforming power, restorative justice seeks to repair the damage, right the wrong, and restore the victim, the offender, and the community. The Church is transformed when it responds to the claims of discipleship by becoming an agent of healing and systemic change.

The UMC has produced curriculum on restorative justice themes entitled *Restorative Justice: Moving Beyond Punishment* (Wray, 2002).

Episcopal

In July 2000, the 73rd General Convention of the Episcopal Church passed the following resolution:

> Resolved . . . that the . . . Episcopal Church embrace the concept of restorative justice for our nation's justice system; and be it further resolved, that the General Convention issue a call to the wider Christian community and other interfaith and nonprofit organizations to join it in urging that our nation's public policies embrace restorative justice, and be it further resolved, that the General Convention affirm that in a just and fair system of social order, one where both forgiveness and mercy are balanced with accountability and restitution, reflecting for us the Baptismal Covenant in seeking and serving Christ in all persons, and striving for justice and peace among all people, and respecting the dignity of every human being.

Through the efforts of the Episcopal Peace Fellowship, the Episcopal Church is working to bring these resolutions to life.

Baptist

The Baptist Peace Fellowship of North America has a restorative justice program offering resource materials and networking among Baptists concerned with our criminal justice system and wanting to move it into the restorative justice paradigm (Hanneman, 2001).

American Baptist

The American Baptist Church USA (ABCUSA) adopted a Statement of Concern (which expresses to American Baptists and the rest of society the opinion of those delegates present on a particular matter) on Restorative Justice at its June 2001 Biennial Meeting. Later that year, the ABCUSA General Board adopted a Resolution on Restorative Justice, which states:

> Restorative justice offers a framework with which to bring a reparative and holistic focus to the center of the criminal justice system. At its core, restorative justice views crime as a violation of people and relationships, and justice as a process that actively works to repair those harmed by crime . . . This process of repairing the harm to the victim has as an equal and parallel goal: the restoration of the offender to the community. This relational approach to justice invites victims, offenders and communities to be actively involved in the justice process.

> Through its Office of Reconciliation Ministries, ABCUSA provides resources to equip churches and individuals to be a mediating presence in the midst of community conflicts, especially conflicts that involve ethnic or cultural differences; offers a basic fourteen-hour workshop offering skills so participants can analyze social conflict, develop transformative listening capacities, and become competent in using a mediation process that can be adapted to different situations. The ABCUSA also works on a variety of other projects, including prison ministries and restorative justice, to help churches work towards social justice and healing, and maintains a liaison with the Baptist Peace Fellowship of North America.

Southern Baptist

The Southern Baptist Women's Missionary Union has chosen restorative justice as the social issue they are addressing during the next two years. Under the title *Project HELP: Restorative Justice*, they offer a variety of resources for study and discussion.

Prison Fellowship

Prison Fellowship International hosts *Restorative Justice Online* as a service of their International Centre for Justice and Reconciliation. Their Website *www.icjr.org* states:

> The purpose of *Restorative Justice Online* is to be a credible, non-partisan source of information on restorative justice. The site is divided into sections for ease of use: The Introduction includes definitions and slideshow presentations about important issues in restorative justice. The Resources section has a searchable, annotated bibliography on restorative justice; annotated links to other sites on restorative justice; and United Nations and Council of Europe documents on restorative topics. The Action section includes slideshow presentations introducing restorative justice and tutorials on restorative justice theory and practice. The Chapel contains articles and other materials from the Judeo-Christian tradition.

Unitarian Universalist

The Unitarian Universalist Association looks at restorative justice in a variety of ways, including using it as a model in cases of clergy sexual misconduct. The concern for the victim and community and the need to repair the harm done is a major focus. They also are developing a restorative justice model in cases of domestic violence.

Ecumenical

The Maine Council of Churches, an ecumenical organization with eight member faith communities, has been working in the Maine criminal justice system for over 15 years. Since 1993 the foundation for their work has been the principles of restorative justice. Their work has been two-fold: systemic involvement to move the criminal justice system into the restorative justice paradigm and providing educational resources to member congregations to inform the general public on criminal justice issues and how they can be addressed through the restorative justice principles.

Successes have occurred on several levels including changes in the law to allow for more restorative possibilities within the system; a focus on restorative justice within the Maine Department of Corrections with the hiring of a victim advocate for the Department of Corrections; support for restorative justice among prosecutors, judges, and some defense attorneys; and the formation of a Victim Offender Mediation Program. The Maine Council of Churches has received a planning grant to study the feasibility of establishing a Restorative Justice Center to coordinate restorative justice activities within the state.

Roman Catholic

Perhaps the faith community with the most comprehensive analysis of crime and criminal justice is the Roman Catholic Church. The statement approved in November 2000 by the nearly 350 bishops of the United States, *Responsibility, Rehabilitation and Restoration: A Catholic Perspective on Crime and Criminal Justice*, is an expansive study of the many issues surrounding crime. The Catholic Church not only has a network of social service agencies (i.e., Catholic Charities) that offer services to people in need, including those impacted by crime, but also has designated significant resources through the Catholic Campaign for Human Development to fund specific programs in this area. The balance of this paper will look at the bishops' study and the projects inspired by it and funded by the Catholic Church.

CATHOLICS EXPAND FOCUS TO NEEDS OF VICTIMS AND COMMUNITY

In *Responsibility, Rehabilitation and Restoration: A Catholic Perspective on Crime and Criminal Justice*, the bishops take a fresh look at the complexities of dealing with crime, victimization, and community safety, placing concern for victims and for communities up front. Not neglected in the document are the perpetrators of crime and society's response to them, but there is a clear shift in addressing the need for community safety and victim assistance. The bishops drew on the experiences of Catholic Charities agencies, their policy staff at the state and local level, pastors in high crime areas and theologians and ethicists.

The result of the study and consultation is the document's emphasis on responsibility and restoration. The overriding message of the statement is: "We will not tolerate the crime and violence that threatens the lives and dignity of our sisters and brothers, and we will not give up on those who have lost their way. We seek both justice and mercy" (USCC, 2000, p. 55). The document is not a simply a condemnation of the current criminal justice system–although it questions many current practices, nor is it a stamp of approval of the status quo–although it recognizes the need for community safety and personal responsibility. Instead it moves into a positive direction by calling for a restorative response to crime.

Responsibility, Rehabilitation and Restoration: A Catholic Perspective on Crime and Criminal Justice is divided into three primary sections: what is currently happening in the criminal justice system, what the Catholic faith and tradition have to say about this, and, based on these realities and this teaching, what society and Catholics ought to do to better respond to the myriad problems created by crime.

To the question, is restorative justice–that is, justice that seeks to heal the victim, restore the offender and bring wholeness to the community–part of the Christian tradition? The answer is an unqualified yes. The whole tradition affirms it, from the Hebrew teaching on shalom (right relationships) to the New Testament's emphasis on love, justice, mercy, and wholeness, to St. Paul's admonition to:

> Bless those who persecute (you), bless and do not curse them. Rejoice with those who rejoice, weep with those who weep. Have the same regard for one another; do not be haughty but associate with the lowly; do not be wise in your own estimation. Do not repay anyone evil for evil; be concerned for what is noble in the sight of all. If possible, on your part, live at peace with all. Beloved, do not look for revenge but leave room for the wrath; for it is written, "Vengeance is mine, I will repay, says the Lord." Rather, "if your enemy is hungry, feed him; if he is thirsty, give him something to drink; for by so doing you will heap burning coals upon his head." Do not be conquered by evil but conquer evil with good. (Romans 12:14-21)

The church has taken seriously the need to help, heal, comfort and restore.

Policy and program suggestions for both society at large and the church are proposed in the statement. Granted that a basic function of the criminal justice system is the protection of society, punishment must be coupled with treatment and, when possible, restitution. Society is called upon to reject simplistic solutions such as "three strikes and you're out" and rigid mandatory sentencing noting that just as the causes of crime are complex so, too, should be our work to fight crime and restore communities. Highlighted, too, is a warning not to treat young offenders as though they are adults. They are not "fully formed in conscience and fully aware of their actions. Placing children in adult jails is a sign of failure, not a solution" (USCC, 2000, p. 28).

It may be helpful to elaborate on the *option for the poor,* a basic principle of Catholic social teaching. It is a response to Jesus' charge to us, "whatsoever you do to the least of these, you do unto me" (Matthew 25: 45), that is, in the poor, we encounter Jesus. Because we are all made in God's image and likeness, and, therefore, each person is sacred and precious in God's eyes, encounters with Jesus through others are possible. But the principle of the option for the poor tells Catholics that it is especially in the poor that we meet Jesus. In a corollary teaching, the Hebrew Scriptures say that a primary measure of society is how it treats the "anaweim"–the widow, the orphan, and the stranger. Why these people? Because they do not have a voice, they are not at the decision making table. Or if they are, they do not need to be listened too (Kammer, 1995).

A significant moral test of any society is how it treats "the least among us." Those imprisoned are certainly of this number. How are we treating those in prison? Should we be putting behind bars so many men and women with substance abuse problems when treatment is needed to help them regain their wholeness and sense of value and worth as human beings? While it is thought necessary to remove from communities those that threaten the lives and safety of those around them, wholesale incarceration for drug and alcohol offenses leads one to question: how well this society is living up to this basic moral test for any society.

Poverty is exacerbated by incarceration because of the loss of income of a father/mother, husband/wife. Further, loss of parental caring through incarceration is particularly hard on children and often continues or begins a cycle of poverty, crime and incarceration for generations. For all of these reasons, a full-scale assault on poverty would serve well the cause of increasing community safety and decreasing crime.

Calling for more serious efforts toward crime prevention and poverty reduction, it is held that extreme poverty and racism often shape American attitudes and policies toward crime and criminal justice. Combating poverty, educating against racism, and supporting families will all help deter crime.

Asserting that we live in a "culture of violence," we attempt to solve some of our most intractable problems with violence. From abortion and the death penalty, to violence on our television and in our gestures, we are a remarkably violent society. Serious efforts to find alternatives to violence, including the violence of incarceration, are desperately needed. Specific policies such as the regulation of handguns and less violence in our movies and television, to broader cultural attitudes such as personal responsibility, less selfishness and individualism, are all necessary to help reduce the amount of violence in the U.S. society.

Victims and their families should be afforded a greater role in the criminal justice process. Highlighting the fact that an offense is not just against the state but also against real people living in the community, it is recognized that society must pay more attention to the physical, emotional and spiritual needs of victims. Rejected, however, is any exploitation of victims to seek more punitive sentences or tougher policies against the perpetrators of crime.

Much more can be done to build on the budding efforts of communities trying new approaches to crime generally recognized as "restorative justice." The shift in emphasis to the victim and the community harmed by the crime rather than just the offense to the state by the perpetrator is fully consistent with the Church's teaching on justice and mercy. The church's social teaching principle of *subsidiarity* comes into clearer focus here.

> Subsidiarity calls for problem solving initially at the community level: family, neighborhood, city, and state. It is only when problems become too large or the common good is clearly threatened that larger institutions are required to help. This principle encourages communities to be more involved. Criminal activity is largely a local issue and, to the extent possible, should have local solutions. Neighborhood-watch groups, community-oriented policing, school liaison officers, neighborhood treatment centers, and local support for ex-offenders all can be part of confronting crime and fear of crime in local communities. (USCC, 2000, p. 25)

Over the past several decades, communities, mostly out of fear of crime, have relegated the responsibility for ensuring safety to government demonstrated in their willingness to build more prisons, put more police on the streets and get tougher on even minor offenses. There were times when the community was intimately involved in confronting the offender, comforting the victim and setting the conditions for the offender to return to the community. The dominant model now, however, is that a crime is against the state with little regard for the needs of the victim or the community. However, true restorative justice should not be seen as soft on crime, because in most instances offenders are called to face the human consequences of their acts to the victims and/or their families. Offenders are also often more willing to accept responsibility and offer restitution when such an approach is pursued.

Recognizing the positive influence that religion can have in the lives of all people, prison officials are urged to support and even encourage inmates to express their religious beliefs and give opportunity for practice. Through chaplaincy programs, the churches have traditionally helped in this endeavor.

Finally, crime must be placed in the context of community. "'Community' is not only a place to live; the word also describes the web of relationships and resources that brings us together and helps us cope with our everyday challenges" (USCC, 2000, p. 44). Crime and its consequences harm the web. In many communities individuals and organizations have confronted violence and restored their communities. Often local churches have organized to fight crime, and many of these efforts are funded by the bishops' Catholic Campaign for Human Development.

WHAT CAN CHURCHES DO?

What can individual people of faith and their churches do to help reduce crime, minister to victims, offenders and their families? How can church institutions use their moral influence to affect policy changes at the local, state and national levels so that the criminal justice system is more reflective of the values of faith communities? Examples from many faith communities have been cited earlier. The following are descriptions of some actions recently instigated by the Catholic Church.

As a result of the document, the bishops' committee, which oversees the work of the Catholic Campaign for Human Development (CCHD), has allocated $1.5 million to help dioceses and other local groups implement some of the policy recommendations found in *Responsibility, Rehabilitation and Restoration: A Catholic Perspective on Crime and Criminal Justice*.

CCHD was founded in 1970 by the U.S. Catholic bishops to significantly reduce poverty in the United States through empowerment of those people affected. The Campaign has provided millions of dollars raised through an annual Sunday collection in all Catholic churches to assist low-income controlled community or church-based organizing projects as they work to improve their neighborhoods and change policies that exacerbate poverty.

Special CCHD grants that are part of the $1.5 million awarded over the past two years are focused on two dozen projects that address significant criminal justice issues. Some of these are described below.

California

Under the auspices of the California Catholic Conference, the public policy voice for the California bishops in Sacramento, and through the experiences of many diocesan detention ministry staff, California lawmakers may soon come to the conclusion that new and more innovative approaches to crime and criminal justice may be necessary.

In October of 2000, the California Catholic Conference's Ad Hoc Committee on Prison Ministry and Corrections produced a report that was presented to the California State Department of Corrections. The report outlined some of the policy steps needed to make the corrections system more humane and more consistent with the values of the Church.

The original charter of the Ad Hoc Committee was to "improve the Church's role in ministering to prisoners, victims and families" (California Catholic Conference, 2000 p. 1). Their report identified issues that must be addressed by the Church and by the state. The potential impact of the activity of the Ad Hoc Committee is great, for California has nearly 160,000 people incarcerated in 33 state prisons, 38 camps, and 10 youth detention facilities.

Many areas are cited in which more effort is required in addressing the pastoral needs of inmates, victims, their families, and more clarity in its role in advocating for social changes to reduce crime and its consequences. The Committee is working to ensure that all Catholic inmates have access to a Catholic chaplain. They have developed uniform screening procedures for chaplain candidates, intensified recruiting efforts, and put in place procedures to ensure that volunteer and paid chaplains are fulfilling the requirements of the job.

In the area of family, programs are being developed that will help alleviate the strain caused by the incarceration of a spouse, including marriage strengthening programs, and other outreach particularly needed because the stigma attached to incarceration often makes families reluctant to seek spiritual, material and emotional assistance from the church. Efforts are underway to work with diocesan peace and justice offices to become more fully aware of the link between incarceration and poverty, urging these offices to work for policy solutions that address poverty, ultimately helping to lower crime and incarceration rates.

Hearing from inmates themselves that there are few opportunities to reconcile with the victims of their crimes, increased attention and more resources are now going to boost efforts such as victim-offender reconciliation programs, and other outreach to victims.

The Ad Hoc Committee has developed a framework to assist dioceses in assessing the needs of newly released men, women and juveniles. Diocesan detention ministry staff, Catholic charities organizations and groups such as the St. Vincent de Paul societies are coordinating these efforts.

Efforts are underway to ensure that the growing number of undocumented immigrants, including those who are detained while they await status hearings, have access to chaplain services. The church is working with the Immigration and Naturalization Service to develop shelter-care alternatives for undocumented minors.

The Committee has urged a moratorium on the use of the death penalty in California in order to study the legal and racial problems that have surfaced in other states. There is an effort to renew ministries to those on death row, including letter writing, praying, and educating the public about the church's teaching on the death penalty.

The California Department of Corrections (CDC) has been asked to re-examine policies to allow for more adequate contact between family members and inmates (and especially between children and their incarcerated mothers). Citing evidence that such contact can be an important motivator to participate in prison rehabilitation programs, the Committee also urges that the CDC offer transportation resources for families of inmates housed far away.

This comprehensive set of recommendations based on the experience of the Ad Hoc Committee's delegations to jails, prisons, and detention facilities is impressive. Further, based on their experience, a handbook for other Catholic groups wanting to send a delegation to a prison has been developed. It outlines the "nuts and bolts" of forming a delegation, coordinating with prison officials, conduct inside the facilities and evaluation of the visit and useful readings and resources in preparation for the visit. This tool has become invaluable to not only engage more Catholics in the area of prison ministry, but because of its thoroughness and step-by-step approach, it has broken down the suspicion and distrust that often accompanies such "fact-finding" missions in the past.

As a culmination of the efforts of the Ad Hoc Committee, the California Catholic Conference, with the assistance of the Archdiocese of Los Angeles and Loyola Marymount University in Southern California, planned a daylong symposium. Its purpose was to offer Catholics and other people of faith an opportunity to explore new ways to assist victims and their families, to reach out to offenders and their families, to build communities that are safe and whole, and to discuss policy changes that will offer real alternatives to the current approaches to crime and criminal justice.

Northern California

Other dioceses have begun the design and dissemination of educational materials about a Catholic approach to crime and criminal justice. Also funded by the Catholic Campaign for Human Development, the Archdiocese of San Francisco is planning a project with the dioceses of Oakland, San Jose, and Santa Rosa, as well as the Sisters of Mercy, to produce a video that will raise awareness among the people of the Catholic parishes of Northern California. The video will help to put a face on the victims and perpetrators of crime; to remind Catholics of their core values, especially human life and human dignity; to explore the inadequacies of the current criminal justice system; to help offenders understand their obligations to make amends to the victims and to help them find ways to turn others away from a life of crime; and to offer concrete ways for parishioners to become engaged in helping victims, offenders and to build the capacity of the church to affect laws that would better reflect the values of restorative justice. The accompanying study guide will familiarize Catholics with the 2000 bishops' statement, and provide a series of reflection questions.

North Carolina

In Chatham County, North Carolina, the Diocese of Raleigh is working to ensure that the growing Hispanic populations have equal access to the justice that is promised by the criminal justice system. Those who serve this immigrant community have found many civil rights violations and inadequate access to police protection that affect both Latino crime victims and those accused of offenses. Local law enforcement agencies have had difficulties in establishing trust in the Latino community stemming from their experience of police in their former countries. In summary, the cultural gap has created numerous problems when the Latino population comes in contact with either the protection or enforcement ends of the legal system. A number of projects to address these issues are underway, including the formation of a new Criminal Justice Advisory Committee. This advisory committee will provide training for criminal justice system personnel to raise awareness of the needs and barriers faced by the new immigrant population, to demonstrate ways to build trust with this community, and to explain the basics of immigration laws. Initially, training will be for law enforcement officers, but will also be extended to others in the system, including judges, public defenders, district attorneys and dispatchers.

With the support of the Orange-Chatham Superior Court Judge, the executive director of the project will participate in the Trial Court Performance Standards Task Force. This task force will gather information about the local court system and make recommendations to the Administrative Office of the Courts for improvements. In addition, the project will also take advantage of a daily live Spanish-language call in talk show and broadcast at least two programs each month related to the criminal justice system. Finally, the project will share information about rights, resources, services, and upcoming gatherings and events in the four area bilingual newspapers.

New Mexico

In 1997, the bishops of New Mexico wrote a pastoral letter challenging the system of criminal justice in their state. Spurred by the ideas and challenges from the U.S. bishops' statement and the special funds from the Catholic Campaign for Human Development, the Archdiocese of Santa Fe is organizing ex-offenders in a project to reintegrate them into society and to educate the Catholic community about restorative justice issues. New Mexico may be in a unique situation; nearly 70% of all incarcerated persons in the state are Catholic; both the incarcerated and the victims are members of the faith community.

To begin the challenge of changing state policies in the area of corrections, Archbishop Michael Sheehan and New Mexico's head of the department of corrections have met to begin to talk about more rehabilitation in prison and to explore partnerships with the Church to reintegrate ex-offenders into society.

Two full-time staff are working for the Archdiocese and have already negotiated a revision of ex-offender eligibility guidelines, developed a mentor training program that is being promulgated jointly between the New Mexico corrections and parish and community representatives, and explored ways for the department and faith communities to collaborate together with probation and parole programs as well as with the departments of labor and health to assist with reintegration issues.

Three mentor teams have been trained and matched with adult ex-offenders who are reintegrating into society. There are 20 youth mentors who have been recruited, trained and matched with youth in detention centers in the Archdiocese. An organizing committee of Catholic Detention Organizing Project oversees the reintegration effort of both adults and youth.

The Project is also working to create a network of parishes to advocate for broader rehabilitation programs and to establish a mentor/mentee relationship between parishes and ex-offenders. A special educational event focused on the 2000 bishops' statement on crime and criminal justice is planned.

Oakland

In the Diocese of Oakland, Catholic Charities of the East Bay will draw on its twenty-two year experience in prison ministry to help reintegrate the nearly 4,000 juveniles who pass through the juvenile justice systems in the two counties that comprise the Diocese of Oakland. Nearly all of these youth come from low-income communities and are at extreme risk of lifelong involvement with violence, and substance abuse stemming from family dysfunction and poverty. Operation New Hope is a program of Catholic Charities that understands how critical it is to try to intervene in the lives of these youths as soon as they are released so they do not continue on a path to crime.

The program operates on five basic principles: (1) any program must start with the assumption that youth parolees are intent on changing their lives; (2) reintegration programs must begin working with the youth several weeks prior to release; (3) knowing that the life that awaits them upon release can be the same one that led to their detention, reintegration programs must provide meaningful alternatives to previous lifestyles; (4) parolees need mentors; (5) reentry programs should involve agencies and individuals from the parolee's community.

Based on these presuppositions, Operation New Hope is seeking support from detention facilities to see the value of starting reentry before reentry actually happens and in building relationships with other institutions within communities to ensure successful reintegration. Beginning with the institutions of the Catholic church, the pilot project will be supported by Catholic Charities of the East Bay and enlist the help of detention ministers from 50 parishes, social justice and welfare to work interns, and six high school youth who have agreed to be trained in peer education and community violence prevention programs. Out of this will come 20 people, the juvenile justice team, who will then be trained in the skills necessary to implement the program. As successful models unfold, more teams will be trained so that eventually no child is left without the opportunity to reintegrate into his or her community and break the cycle of offense-incarceration-release.

National

The Catholic Campaign for Human Development has also funded a project aimed at facilitating a dialogue among national ecumenical interfaith groups. National staff from a variety of Christian denominations, including Roman Catholic, Evangelical Lutherans, United Methodists, Mennonite, Episcopalians, United Churches of Christ, Baptists, Quakers, as well as representatives from the Jewish and Muslim faiths, among others, will be convened. The goal of the Interfaith Coordination Committee for Restorative Justice Policies is to develop itself into a broad-based coalition of faith groups that will work with its member communities and like-minded secular coalitions to develop and promote criminal and juvenile justice reform based on restorative justice principles.

It is hoped that the groups can come to common agreement on principles of restorative justice and then apply those principles to specific policy initiatives aimed at the reformation of state and federal approaches to crime and criminal justice. Through education materials, grassroots organizing, advocacy skills training, and by coordinating a common agenda, the Interfaith Coordinating Committee hopes to create a united voice so that society's approach to crime can be more reflective of the core values of all faith groups.

CONCLUSION

Many faith communities have embraced the principles of restorative justice, finding its biblical roots appealing and consistent with their mission, and its opportunity for healing the wounds caused by crime for all its victims very attractive. They are reaching out increasingly to educate and to motivate their congregations and others. Putting these principles into practice requires resources that are not always readily available, but as has been amply shown in this paper, churches have found ways to become significant players in restorative justice education and action. By sponsoring VORPs, participating in community conferencing groups, advocating for justice, volunteering in prison ministries, opening their buildings to groups serving offenders or victims, faith communities have done remarkable work. With the "charitable choice" provision of the PRWORA, new funding partnerships with the Federal government offer hope for an expanded role for church sponsored restorative justice programs.

REFERENCES

California Catholic Conference. (2000). *Report to the California Department of Corrections.* Sacramento: California Catholic Conference.

Hanneman, E. (2001). *Seeking shalom: Why our current criminal justice system doesn't work and what every Christian needs to know about how to fix it.* Charlotte. Baptist Peace Fellowship of North America (*www.bpfna.org*).

Kammer, F. (1995). *Salted with fire: Spirituality for the faith justice journey.* New York/Mahwah, NJ: Paulist Press.

Mackey, V. & Shadle, C. *Justice or "just desserts?" An adult study of the restorative justice approach.* Presbyterian Distribution Service. 1-800-524-2612.

Personal Responsibility and Work Opportunity Reconciliation Act of 1996, P.L. 104-193, 110 stat.2105.

Resolution on Restorative Justice. Adopted by the General Board of the American Baptist Churches. November 2001.

United States Conference of Catholic Bishops. *New American Bible* as posted on *http://www.usccb.org/nab/bible.*

United States Catholic Conference. (2000). *Responsibility, rehabilitation and restoration: A Catholic perspective on crime and criminal justice.* Washington: United States Catholic Conference.

Van Ness, D. & Strong, K. H. (1997). *Restoring justice.* Cincinnati: Anderson Publishing Co. 9-10.

Wolterstorff, N. (1999). The contours of justice: An ancient call for shalom. In Lampman, L. & M. Shattuck (Eds.), *God and the victim: Theological reflections on evil, victim-*

ization, justice, and forgiveness. Grand Rapids: Wm. B Eerdmans Publishing Co. & Neighbors Who Care. 113.

Wray, H. & Hutchison. P. (2002). *Restorative justice: Moving beyond punishment.* Includes *Study Guide* by B. Connelly. General Board of Global Ministries, United Methodist Church.

Zehr, H. J. (1990). *Changing lenses: A new focus for crime and justice.* Scottsdale, PA: Herald Press.

The Practice and Efficacy
of Restorative Justice

Kay Pranis

SUMMARY. Beginning with an exploration of the importance of understanding the power of questions, this paper examines the question, "Does it work?" regarding restorative justice as a philosophy and a set of practices based on that philosophy. The paper identifies problems in the dominant retributive philosophical paradigm for responding to crime that the philosophy of restorative justice resolves. The author describes the practices of restorative justice in criminal justice as well as other contexts and presents evidence of effectiveness in achieving restorative outcomes. The paper discusses challenges and limitations in restorative practices. *[Article copies available for a fee from The Haworth Document Delivery Service: 1-800-HAWORTH. E-mail address: <docdelivery@haworthpress.com> Website: <http://www.HaworthPress.com> © 2004 by The Haworth Press, Inc. All rights reserved.]*

KEYWORDS. Restorative justice, effectiveness and restorative justice, restorative practices, challenges and restorative justice

---

Kay Pranis is a former restorative planner, Minnesota Department of Corrections, 1450 Energy Park Drive, Suite 200, St. Paul, MN 55108.

[Haworth co-indexing entry note]: "The Practice and Efficacy of Restorative Justice." Pranis, Kay. Co-published simultaneously in *Journal of Religion & Spirituality in Social Work* (The Haworth Social Work Practice Press, an imprint of The Haworth Press, Inc.) Vol. 23, No. 1/2, 2004, pp. 133-157; and: *Criminal Justice: Retribution vs. Restoration* (ed: Eleanor Hannon Judah, and Rev. Michael Bryant) The Haworth Social Work Practice Press, an imprint of The Haworth Press, Inc., 2004, pp. 133-157. Single or multiple copies of this article are available for a fee from The Haworth Document Delivery Service [1-800-HAWORTH, 9:00 a.m. - 5:00 p.m. (EST). E-mail address: docdelivery@haworthpress.com].

http://www.haworthpress.com/web/JRSSW
© 2004 by The Haworth Press, Inc. All rights reserved.
Digital Object Identifier: 10.1300/J377v23n01_08

Restorative justice has emerged as a different framework for guiding responses to crime at all levels of the criminal justice system. Howard Zehr (2002) identifies three concepts as pillars of this framework: (1) Restorative justice focuses on harm. (2) Wrongs or harms result in obligations. (3) Restorative justice promotes engagement or participation. Restorative justice, then, encompasses responses to crime that move toward understanding, acknowledging and repairing harm. Achieving understanding, acknowledgment and repair requires direct participation of victims, offenders and affected communities in the process of justice. Since harm is the central problem in a restorative framework, restorative justice requires a response that does no deliberate further harm.

In the restorative framework mutual responsibility is the loom on which the fabric of community is woven. Crime represents a failure of responsibility, clearly on the part of the offender and sometimes on the part of the larger community. Restorative justice aims to re-establish mutual responsibility. As interest in restorative justice grows there is an increasing need to assess the effectiveness of this framework in moving communities toward the goal of safety and harmony.

THE POWER OF QUESTIONS–
ASKING THE RIGHT QUESTIONS

The framing of this article, suggested several questions to be answered: Does restorative justice work? If so why and how? When is it appropriate and when not? When has it worked and why? These questions seem straightforward and obvious but they are, in fact, very complicated, requiring analysis in themselves before they are answered. What do we mean by "work"? What are the assumptions behind the questions we ask? What is it we are trying to get at with our questions?

Restorative justice practice recognizes that the question you ask dramatically impacts the intervention that will follow. For instance, when you change the question from, "What should we do to this offender because of the harm he/she did?" to "What should this offender do to make amends for the harm he/she caused?," an entirely different direction in the intervention follows. The shape of our questions determines the shape of the answers to a particular problem.

In a daylong seminar on the overrepresentation of African Americans in Minnesota prisons, one small discussion group was asked to respond to the question, "How is Minnesota so successful in keeping white people out of prison?" At first some participants laughed and thought perhaps it was a facetious question. It was not. It was a serious question. When the group began to answer that question, the discussion provided a very different direction for action than would have emerged in answer to the question, "Why is Minnesota locking up so many African Americans?"

An entire field of study, Appreciative Inquiry, has emerged from the recognition that the way we frame the question has enormous implications for what answers will emerge to shape actions that have real life consequences (Hammond, 1996). Therefore, the questions we choose and the way we understand those questions is very important. The questions we ask are often not neutral. It is a core premise of qualitative research that assumptions are embedded in our questions that are shaped by our values and beliefs (Lofland & Lofland, 1995; Patton, 1990). Examining those assumptions and the underlying values can help clarify how we are using questions and where particular questions might lead us.

Analysis of restorative justice and its practices raises several layers of relevant questions: questions about restorative justice as a philosophy (Van Ness & Strong, 2001; Braithwaite & Petit, 1990) and questions about the design and implementation of restorative justice practices in relation to that philosophy (Bazemore & Schiff, 2001). Within the practices questions are an important tool in prompting dialog among participants about particular events. Asking the right questions–questions that assist individuals or groups in accessing their own wisdom and in reflecting from a posture of seeking positive outcomes–is essential to each of these layers.

Rethinking the Question: Does It Work?

One of the most commonly asked questions about restorative justice is, "Does it work?" It's a natural question, because people want to know if an effort is worth putting energy into, yet it can be a misleading question if we are not clear about whether we are talking about restorative justice as a philosophy and guiding vision, or whether we are talking about the practices that put that vision into practice. The question, "Does it work?" usually asks for quantitative evidence. A philosophy or guiding vision is chosen based on a sense of deep inner truth and does not limit it to that which can be proven by evidence. A philosophy can express our hopes and aspirations, not just our current reality. Choosing our philosophy matters. The world is not an objective reality that remains the same regardless of what we believe (Kuhn, 1962). To a large degree our beliefs shape the world we create with our actions and our energy. Choosing a positive vision contributes to creating a more positive world.

Does Restorative Justice Work as a Philosophy?

So, let's ask the question, "Does it work?" of restorative justice as a philosophy and guiding vision for every aspect of how we respond to harm. What do we expect from a philosophy? We expect that it guide us in understanding how life works and in being intentional about identifying the values we wish to live by and then figuring out how to make them operational. We ask it to give us clear direction about how to conduct ourselves, even in very difficult circumstances. What do we expect of a vision? We expect that it inspires, that it describes a world that we would want to live in, that it draws out our capacities, that it aligns separate individuals in a common quest or endeavor. In the case of a paradigm shift from a current dominant philosophy to a new philosophy, we expect the new philosophy to resolve persistent problems in the prevailing philosophy (Bazemore, 2001).

Does restorative justice as a philosophy and guiding vision meet these expectations? Restorative justice appears remarkably successful as a philosophy and guiding vision. Restorative justice sets out a clear set of values to shape our actions. As a philosophy, it assists us in understanding the concrete, personal harm of crime and its effect on relationships and community. It also helps us design pathways for repair and healing of those negative impacts. It provides reasonably clear direction for our conduct. While not prescriptive about strategies, restorative justice is clear about the goals of actions and the value-constraints that limit actions. Practitioners may disagree about some specific approaches and their degree of alignment with restorative values, but there is a high level of agreement about what core practices look like and what makes them restorative (McCold, 2000; Bazemore, 2000; Walgrave, 2000).

As a philosophy for a new paradigm, restorative justice does resolve serious dilemmas of the prevailing paradigm of justice. The criminal justice system is under great stress and pressure to demonstrate its effectiveness. Both the public and professionals within the system register high levels of dissatisfaction. In the current paradigm, the criminal justice system faces the following dilemmas:

- lack of clarity about the purpose of sentencing;
- contradictory impulses between punishment and rehabilitation;

- victim frustration and alienation;
- public expectation that the criminal justice system will control crime;
- failure of increasing punishment to change behavior;
- skyrocketing costs of punishment;
- failure to integrate social justice with criminal justice; and
- widespread system overload (Pranis, 1992).

Despite heroic efforts of dedicated professionals and high levels of spending over the past two decades, relatively little progress has been made on these problems within the dominant paradigm. Restorative justice as a philosophy resolves these persistent problems.

Lack of Clarity About the Purpose of Sentencing

Restorative justice establishes the purpose of sentencing, above all else, as repair of the harm done to the victim, to the offender himself, and to the community, including the harm of losing a sense of safety within the community. Other purposes may be served but are secondary.

Punishment versus Rehabilitation

Restorative justice replaces the focus on punishment, measured by how much pain is inflicted, with a focus on accountability, measured by taking responsibility and taking action to repair the harm. This kind of accountability, while often painful, supports growth and healing and does not conflict with rehabilitation (Bazemore, Nissen, & Dooley, 2000; Braithwaite, 2001).

Victim Frustration

Restorative justice prioritizes victim involvement, victim choice, and sensitivity to victims' concerns throughout the process, including post adjudication. Without a victim perspective, we cannot be sure of exactly what the harm was and what would be helpful to repair the harm. Victim satisfaction is a high priority in restorative justice (Achilles & Zehr, 2001; Umbreit, 1999).

Failure of Increasing Punishment to Change Behavior

Restorative justice is not premised on the assumption that punishment will change behavior and does not rely on producing results through punishment.

Public Expectation that the Criminal Justice System Will Solve the Problem of Crime

We know that actions of the criminal justice system have limited impact on the crime rate, yet our paradigm suggests that the criminal justice system has a primary role in changing crime rates. We are unable to deliver what the model seems to promise. Restorative justice has a goal of reparation and measures outcomes based on the question: "To what degree has the harm been repaired and power relationships put right?" In restorative justice crime control is clearly identified as a function of community and government partnerships that include criminal justice but extend well beyond criminal justice.

Skyrocketing Cost of Punishment

Restorative justice requires fewer investments in punishment since the system is measured, not by how much punishment is inflicted, but by how much reparation and healing are achieved.

Failure to Integrate Social Justice with Criminal Justice

This is perhaps the most serious failing of our present system. Restorative justice clearly defines a relationship between social justice and criminal justice. The community is held responsible for community "shalom." Individuals are held responsible for their behavior. A bad environment does not excuse individuals of responsibility for causing harm to others, but at the same time the community is held accountable for promoting community peace, including social justice. The community is expected to take responsibility for supporting victims, helping offenders take responsibility, and addressing underlying causes of crime. The community is not allowed to simply banish people and expect someone else to deal with the behavior as though the community had no part in creating the problem. Restorative justice integrates individual and social responsibility in a coherent conceptual framework (Pranis, 2001).

System Overload

Responding to crime through repair of harm, problem-solving through conflict resolution, and involving families and communities spreads the workload to multiple stakeholders, not just the criminal justice system, and engages all these stakeholders in a commitment of finding workable solutions (Braithwaite, 2001). As a paradigm shift, restorative justice helps us understand differently the problems that are intractable in the current paradigm and provides direction for resolving those problems.

As a vision restorative justice has energized a grassroots movement across the globe in the face of one of the most powerful and entrenched systems in the modern world, the criminal justice system. With very little money and a prevailing public discourse in the media and politics that is exactly the opposite of restorative justice, this vision is nonetheless moving powerfully forward. Many criminal justice professionals speak of being reenergized and invigorated by this vision in a way they have not experienced in the past twenty-five years of their careers. Restorative justice as a vision has brought together people who would never have imagined working together–inner city residents with criminal justice professionals, former victims with former offenders, European-Americans with Hmong-Americans, judges with community members, gang members with police, conservatives with progressives, atheists with Christians. Restorative justice as a vision has provided common ground for a wide variety of perspectives and worldviews.

As a vision restorative justice has drawn out skills, energy and passion from people who previously saw no place for themselves in responding to crime. Energy to address the problems of crime and conflict in our communities is coming from many outside the justice system, creating a sense of shared ownership of the problems and the solutions. As a movement with no clear center, singular leadership or national infrastructure, restorative justice has a remarkable sense of coherence across cultures, organizations, and sectors. Restorative justice is moving organically and is not dependent upon charismatic leadership or traditional structural legitimacy for its sense of authenticity and purpose.

Restorative justice is clearly inspiring, describing a world people want to live in, drawing out potentials, capacity, and aligning endeavors in a common quest. As a vision, it works.

DO THE PRACTICES OF RESTORATIVE JUSTICE WORK?

Now, let's examine the question, "Does it work?" as it might be applied to restorative justice as a cluster of practices that put the philosophy of restorative justice into effect. What do we expect of our practices? What would be the characteristics of "working" for practices intended to move toward this vision? We expect our practices to be consistent with the values and direction embedded in our philosophy. We expect our practices to result in changes that move us closer to the world described by our vision. To "work" as a practice is both a means and an ends question. The practice must not only produce results that move toward the vision, but it must also produce those in a way that does not violate the philosophy. Otherwise the practice is not working to operationalize that philosophy.

The vision of restorative justice describes a world in which harm has been repaired for victims, offenders, and communities and a world in which those who cause harm take responsibility and contribute to the repair. It also describes a world in which power relationships are put into proper balance. So our practices should result in victims, offenders and communities who are in some way in a better position than they were before the restorative intervention. Our practices should have offenders involved in repair of harm to the victim and the community, and they should support offenders in taking responsibility for their actions.

The following characteristics describe practices that are "working" to move us toward that vision (Pranis, 1994):

- The practice provides opportunity for increased involvement of victims.
- The practice produces repair of the harm of the crime for victims to the degree possible.
- The practice increases offender understanding of the harm of the behavior to the victim, the community, and the self.
- The practice encourages offenders to take responsibility for the harm done.
- The practice actively engages the offender in repairing harm to the victim and the community.
- The practice produces repair of the harm of the crime for the community to the degree possible.
- The practice involves community members and encourages the community to take a share of responsibility for repairing harm and managing behavior in the community.
- The practice results in changes that will reduce the likelihood of the crime happening again.
- The practice increases the capacity for self-regulation in individuals and communities.

It is not necessary for a restorative practice to have all of those characteristics. It must, however, have at least one of them and must not in its implementation undermine any of the others.

A broad overarching question for any specific intervention is: Does the intervention leave the community stronger than it was before the crime happened? (Pranis, 2001).

In addition to the characteristics listed above, it is necessary to examine how the practice is carried out, the "means" question. If the process of responding to an offender is humiliating or demeaning, the outcome is unlikely to be a respectful attitude by the offender. If the process of responding to a victim is patronizing or discounts the victim's voice, the outcome is unlikely to be the recovery of personal power (Pranis, 1997). Are the means consistent with the desired ends? Is the practice carried out with respect toward and acknowledgement of the inherent human dignity in everyone?

WHAT ARE THE PRACTICES?
WHAT DOES RESTORATIVE JUSTICE
LOOK LIKE ON THE GROUND?

An eighty-year-old woman, disturbed by noises in the middle of the night, discovered a masked man wielding a crow bar attempting to force his way into her house. She called the police and they found the perpetrator nearby. The victim accepted the opportunity to meet face to face with the young man, who had pled guilty to the offense, to tell him how the crime had affected her life and to participate in deciding how he should make amends. The offender also agreed to participate. A trained facilitator met with both parties separately to hear their stories and explain the process. When the parties came together the elderly woman described the emotional trauma, which was heightened by the recent loss of her husband. The offender apologized and agreed to pay the costs of an alarm system for her as well as the cost of replacing the door. He promised the woman that he would not do it again. Some months later the woman read in the local paper that the same young man had burglarized a local business. She called the facilitator and asked to meet with the young man again. She was very upset that the young man had not kept his word to her. With some trepidation the young man agreed to meet with her. At their second meeting the elderly woman repeated again and again, "How am I going to know you won't do this again? How am I going to know you won't do this again? How am I going to know you won't do this again?" Finally, they agreed that he would call her on the phone every week to reassure her that he was not getting into trouble. Two years later he was still crime free since that incident–the longest time he had gone without committing a new offense.

Because restorative justice is a philosophy to guide all activities in response to crime, it is not a fixed set of practices. However, there are several practices that have emerged under this philosophy that exemplify the philosophy and are often the core of efforts to build a more restorative system. The practices which bring victims and offenders or victims, offenders and community members together in a facilitated dialog to determine what is needed to repair the harm and build a better future are those generally associated with restorative justice. Many other practices, by working with just offenders or just victims, also work toward the vision of restorative justice by supporting victims, involving offenders in repairing harm, increasing offender awareness of responsibility or other restorative goals but may not involve a face-to-face dialog between the victim and the offender.

FACE-TO-FACE RESTORATIVE PRACTICES– VARIOUS MODELS

Victim Offender Dialog/Mediation/Conferences

The classic victim-offender mediation model involves a victim and an offender meeting in a facilitated process in which each party has the opportunity to talk about what happened and ask questions. Emotions are allowed to be expressed within a respectful atmosphere. Most mediations result in a consensus agreement about activities the offender will undertake to meet the needs or expectations of the victim.

Restorative Group Conferences

This model is based on the family group conference introduced in the U.S. in 1994 from Australia. It is an adaptation of a traditional Maori process for resolving community problems. In this process the victim, victim supporters, offender, offender supporters and a facilitator engage in a dialog to explore what happened, how each of them has been affected, and what needs to happen to make things as right as possible. The facilitator may use a script to guide the dialog. Every participant has an opportunity to speak to the issues and the agreement. Expressing emotions is encouraged. Again, agreements about the obligations for the offender are by consensus of all participants.

Peacemaking Circles

Based on American Indian talking circles, the peacemaking circle process involves the victim, victim supporters, offender, offender supporters and interested community members in a structured dialog about what happened, why it happened, what the impact is, and what is needed to repair the harm and prevent it from happening again. Participants sit in a circle without tables or other furniture. An object, called a talking piece, circulates in order among participants who speak only when they are holding the talking piece. The use of the talking piece reduces the role of the facilitator and eliminates cross talk or interruptions because the talking piece designates who may speak while all others listen. The process may involve separate circles for the victim and offender before all parties are brought together to determine an action plan to address the issues raised in the process. By consensus the circle may develop the sentence for the offender and may also stipulate responsibilities of community members and justice officials as part of the agreement.

Community Boards or Panel

In this model a small number of trained community members meet with an offender to talk about what happened, how it has affected the victim and the community and to determine activities to be undertaken by the offender to address restorative goals. Some panels involve victims, others get input from the victim.

These models are relatively fluid and are continuously being adapted to meet particular circumstances or to take advantage of a technique learned from another model. Some restorative group conferencing models include community members who were not directly attached to the event. Some victim offender mediation sessions encourage participants to bring supporters and allow them to speak at some point in the process. Some group conferencing programs use a talking piece for the agreement phase of the process but not for other phases.

All of these processes require admission by the offender of the charge. Victim participation is always voluntary and offender participation is typically voluntary or represents some level of willingness relative to other options. These processes can be used for determining obligations of offenders at many different points of the justice system: informal diversion, formal diversion, post-charge pre-adjudication, and post adjudication as part of the sentence. The peacemaking circle process can be used for the adjudication itself as a sentencing circle. These processes are also used post conviction as a part of healing or as a part of reintegration into the community after a period of incarceration. In the United States referral to a restorative process by the justice system is optional.

There is great variety among states and localities in the implementation process and choice of models. In some states a model may be relatively standardized and in others each group or community designs its own unique approach consistent with the philosophy of restorative justice. In Vermont community boards, initiated by the state Department of Corrections, are in every county and the model is similar throughout the state. In Colorado a common group conferencing model is used in many communities around the state, but each program is locally initiated. In Minnesota programs have developed from grass roots organizing around the philosophy and vary considerably in the specifics of implementation. These face-to-face programs have been initiated by a wide variety of people—probation officers, judges, prosecutors, community activists, victims, police, faith communities, and nonprofits.

In addition to the use of these face-to-face processes at the front end of the system, all of these processes can be used when an offender is returning to the community after serving a period of incarceration. Reintegration into the community is always a critical time for the community and the offender and is often a difficult time for the victim as well. These processes allow an opportunity for dialog about fears, concerns and hopes, provide input into conditions which might be a part of the release plan, and can develop support plans to maximize the possibility of successful re-entry so that new victims are not created.

NON FACE-TO-FACE RESTORATIVE PRACTICES

In many cases it will not be appropriate or feasible to have a face-to-face meeting between the victim and offender. However, efforts toward the goals of repairing harm to the victim, offender and community and encouraging offenders to take responsibility are still possible and are clearly within the restorative vision. These practices often involve working just with the victim or with the offender. Additionally, offenders alone can repair not all harm. Often community or government resources are needed in addition to offender efforts, so offenders may not be involved at all in some restorative practices.

Victim services provide information and support to victims, acknowledging the harm the victim has experienced and reconnecting the victim to the community. Victim reparation funds help repair the financial harm to victims. Community service, if designed to be work that is valued by the community, gives the offender a sense of accomplishment and involves the offender in repairing harm to the community. Creative community service projects involving inmates in institutions have given them a way to repair harm to the community while locked up. Restitution involves the offender in direct repair of the harm to the victim. Apologies and apology letters are restorative if they are sincere and clearly take responsibility for the harm done. They help repair harm by restoring a sense of what is right and wrong and affirming that the victim is not responsible for the hurt or loss. As in any restorative practice the victim has a choice about whether to receive an apology.

Several restorative practices bring victims and offenders together, but not the victims and offenders of the same incident, so they are not face-to-face in the same sense as the practices described above. Victim impact classes or panels for offenders on probation or in prison increase offender understanding of the impact of their behavior, an important component of taking responsibility. These classes or panels also provide an opportunity for victims to tell their story, an important part of the healing process for many victims. Victim offender groups, generally involving victims and offenders impacted by serious crimes and meeting weekly for 10-12 weeks in a prison, provide opportunities for offenders to learn about the impact of victimization in an even deeper way than the impact classes. Similarly, they provide victims with an opportunity to share their story in a more personal process.

Taking responsibility and making amends, core components of the restorative vision, are often part of treatment programs or cognitive skills programs. Consequently, many of these programs contribute to restorative goals as long as the means of achieving those goals are consistent with restorative values. Any practice that diminishes the core self of the offender or is disrespectful of human dignity would not be restorative.

Restorative practice for professionals in the justice system may be as ordinary as carrying the values of restorative justice into all interactions with offenders and victims. It may be answering the phone with compassion and patience when an angry victim is calling about the case, or it may be routinely asking questions of the offender to prompt offender awareness such as: Who was harmed by your actions? What could you do to make it right?

The involvement of community volunteers in victim services or programs to support offenders making amends or making changes in their lives is also a restorative practice. Volunteer assistance to victims and offenders reconnects them to the community fabric. One of the harms of crime is the disconnection and isolation that result from crime for both victims and offenders. By giving of themselves, volunteers help mend the tear in the community fabric caused by the crime.

Restorative Practices in Justice Systems Management

Restorative practices encompass more than the ways that professionals or community members might work with victims and offenders. Very important management practices and infrastructure within organizations support personnel in implementing restorative practices in their direct work with offenders or victims. Restorative management practices include training staff in restorative justice, job descriptions that prioritize restorative justice, policies that support restorative goals and performance measurement systems that give weight to expectations consistent with restorative philosophy. For example, when an offender owes money for fines, fees and restitution, which is paid first? Systemic restorative practice puts the restitution first (Maloney, Bazemore, & Hudson, 2001).

Restorative Practices Beyond the Justice System

Everything described above in restorative practices relates to the criminal justice system. These practices also have application in many other settings. A model of punishment for wrongdoing similar to the justice system is common in schools, workplaces, communities and families. Because all the same problems with the model arise in those settings, the philosophy of restorative justice has moved beyond the criminal justice system to other sectors where people are searching for a more constructive way to respond to harm—a way that does no further harm and that seeks learning and long-term resolution.

The Minnesota Department of Children, Families and Learning promotes restorative measures in K-12 schools as an alternative to suspension or expulsion and as a classroom management tool to prevent small problems from becoming major flare-ups (Karp & Breslin, 2001). On several college campuses restorative practices are an alternative to the traditional discipline process. Several social service organizations and a juvenile corrections facility have begun using group conferencing and peacemaking circles in the workplace to deal with staff conflict or performance problems. A recent international conference on restorative practices offered an intensive training and workshops on using restorative practices in the workplace. In an Oregon apartment complex, a planned eviction was averted by using a peacemaking circle for the problem tenant and other tenants to work through the issues prompting the proposed eviction. In many settings outside the justice system, restorative practices are being used to respond to conflict or harm by engaging those most impacted in working out a resolution that repairs the harm where possible and moves toward healing for all parties.

Personal Restorative Practices

In the author's own experience and that of many of her colleagues, the work in restorative justice, especially the focus on values, calls for inner reflection and inner work as much as it calls for helping others. The personal and the professional do not separate into distinct boxes. They are inextricably intertwined, offering a way to make our lives more holistic and integrated in all aspects. When we make mistakes or hurt someone, it is important for us to model the process of taking responsibility, hearing how our behavior hurt that person, making amends and making changes necessary to prevent it from happening again. We are all accountable for paying attention to how our behavior impacts others. Restorative justice is not just about a group of people that we set apart with the label of "offender" or the people they hurt. It's about all of us.

DO THESE PRACTICES "WORK"
AS WAYS TO MOVE TOWARD THIS VISION?

The face-to-face practices are designed to increase victim involvement, produce repair of harm, increase offender understanding, encourage offenders to take responsibility and actively involve offenders in repairing the harm, the characteristics identified earlier for practices that "work." Research results indicate that implementation is achieving these goals.

Multiple research studies on victim offender mediation and family group conferencing demonstrate high levels of victim satisfaction, high levels of offender satisfaction and increased payment of restitution compared to court ordered restitution. A meta-analysis examining 22 control group studies of 35 individual restorative justice programs (26 youth, 9 adult) concluded that compared to victims who participated in the traditional justice system, victims who participated in restorative processes were significantly more satisfied and that offenders in restorative justice programs were significantly more likely to complete restitution agreements (Latimer, Dowden, & Muise, 2001). The meta-analysis also found reduced recidivism rates for the restorative justice programs.

Umbreit, Coates and Voss (2002), in a review of 63 studies of restorative justice conferencing in 5 countries (46 studies of victim offender mediation, 13 family group conferencing studies and 4 assessments of peacemaking circles), found remarkably consistent levels of victim and offender satisfaction with conferencing strategies, increased likelihood that restitution contracts would be paid and crime reduction for a significant number of offenders who are involved in restorative conferencing approaches.

A qualitative study of a community circle program in a suburban community found that victims in the circle process felt supported by the community and welcomed the opportunity to participate in the justice process (Coates, Umbreit, & Voss, 2000). The typical case in this program was a pre-charge juvenile misdemeanor referred by the police. In the study every circle participant was able to point out at least one important outcome of the circle. The most important outcomes were: offenders accepting responsibility and being accountable, addressing future relations between the victim and the offender, opportunity to express feelings and awareness of support from the community. The study also found an unusual willingness of volunteers to contribute hours and hours to the work of the circle. "Council participants have strengthened their own sense of being part of a community and of sharing responsibility for what happens in its boundaries" (p. 74).

Research on victim offender mediation and dialog in crimes of severe violence consistently shows high levels of satisfaction and perceptions that the process was helpful on the part of both victims and offenders (Umbreit, Coates, & Voss, 2001). Effects of the mediation session for victims included feeling heard, experiencing less control of offender over them, reduced fear, increased trust in relationships with others, seeing the offender as a person rather than a monster, a sense of peace, reductions in suicidal feelings and release from anger (Roberts, 1995).

A study to determine the effectiveness of the Hollow Water First Nation's holistic healing program, a circle process for sexual abuse victims and offenders, concludes that the program saved over $3 million in justice costs over a ten-year period, in addition to improving economic, cultural and social sustainability of the community (Couture, Parker, Couture, & Laboucane, 2001). Recidivism in that program is approximately two percent.

These are the results called for in the vision. If implemented in ways consistent with the values (respect, voluntariness, equal voice), then these face-to-face practices do successfully operationalize the philosophy. They work.

The non face-to-face practices listed above are identified as restorative based on whether they fit one or more of the characteristics identified for practices that "work," so by definition they can serve restorative ends. However, for many of these practices, such as victim services, restitution or community service, research based on specifically restorative outcomes has not been conducted. Some seem intuitively obvious. For instance, restitution clearly repairs some of the harm to the victim and thus "works" on that dimension of restorative justice, if its implementation is consistent with restorative values. Without research, though, questions remain about whether the victim perceives restitution as repair of the harm. In a restorative framework the people directly impacted determine the efficacy of an intervention. Much work remains to be done in assessing effectiveness of these practices in achieving a restorative vision.

ANOTHER LOOK AT THE QUESTION: DOES IT WORK?

This paper has addressed the question of "Does it work?" as it arises in the current paradigm, a paradigm based on the assumption of objective knowledge that must be validated in rational processes. However, restorative justice posits a different set of assumptions based on interrelatedness. In interrelated world knowledge is not an objective entity with an existence on its own. Knowledge is always in a context and rational processes are not the only way of gaining or demonstrating knowledge. The restorative paradigm requires that we explore other ways of looking at questions and knowledge and that we maintain some awareness of when we are using the old paradigm to discuss the new paradigm.

In the academic and professional fields, the question "Does it work?" is given great weight and primacy. The question is typically asked as though we have a clear consensus about what "works" means. But as we have seen it is not a transparent question. And it may not be as important as we have assumed in the way we are currently asking it. The author's experience in public speaking to very diverse groups in many different communities across the country is that lay community members rarely ask "Does it work?" when restorative philosophy and restorative practices are described to them. They more frequently ask, "Why aren't you already doing it that way?"

For many a restorative approach is common sense and does not require proof–just as many aspects of our life do not require proof. We don't ask for proof that we should eat when we are hungry or that we should sleep when we are tired. Some people don't need proof that, when harm happens, we should focus our response on repairing the harm. And many don't need proof to know that bringing people together in a safe, respectful, reflective process to speak truth and listen deeply will make the community healthier and safer.

Rhea Miller, in her book "Cloudhand, Clenched Fist" (1996), writes about paradigm shifts and an expanded understanding of how we know what we know. Knowledge is not just about facts that arise from the experience of another (normal science), but about the relationship those facts have to our own experience. External "proof," if not resonant with our own truth, is not very compelling. The authenticity and authority of an idea arises from the collective and individual experiences of a group. It cannot simply be bestowed by the pronouncement of an expert. "Does it work?" as a primary, driving question arises in the context of normal science in the old paradigm. In a paradigm shift, great caution must be exercised in using the questions of the old paradigm to determine validity of the new paradigm.

> When a community can draw on and trust its own inner resources to discover the validity of a new paradigm, the community is liberated from bondage to old embedded, fixated ways of being in the world. The community is then able to embrace the creativity of chaos, the possibilities of dreams. People are empowered to imagine new ways of being, to problem-solve on a deep level. (p. 60)

What *do* we ask about our practices to create a feedback loop of information that will support learning, growth and improved practice in moving toward a restorative vision? In "Ethics for the New Millennium," the Dalai Lama (1999) suggests that ethical actions are those that support the well-being of others. We cannot know what is ethical without paying attention to how it will impact others, and we cannot know how our actions impact others without asking them. So, perhaps, for ethical practice, the first and foremost question is: What is the impact of these interventions on the lives of real people from their perspective? And when we get the answer to that question, we ask further: Is that what they want and what we intended? The answers to these questions can guide us as we move forward.

HOW IS THE PHILOSOPHY AND PRACTICE MOVING IN THE U.S.?

For the most part the restorative justice movement in the U.S. has been fueled by individual commitment and passion engaged voluntarily. The federal government has provided important support through national training and the development of a cohort of trainers across the country, but the federal government has not actively promoted restorative justice. A few states like Vermont in its adult corrections system and Pennsylvania in its juvenile system have mandated restorative practices across the state. In most states the development of restorative practices is discretionary and is undertaken by those who are willing to commit extra time and energy to follow a vision. The initiative for restorative justice approaches has come from a variety of places–faith communities, neighborhood organizations, the judiciary, probation, police, victims services, corrections and various levels of government, including city, county and state.

Legislative action and statutory changes have not played a large role in the development and growth of restorative practices. Statutes have been enacted in some states, but they are often reactive rather than proactive. Government support at the state and federal level has generally been through executive branch agencies. In Minnesota, where nearly every model of restorative practice has been implemented, there was no enabling legislation to begin restorative practices. Implementation has been regarded as within the discretion of existing statutes. After programs were already in place, a definition of restorative programs was put into statute to ensure that newly created grant monies would be properly allocated. In some cases, such as Vermont, statutory change was necessary to create options other than prison and probation, but leadership in that policy change came from the Department of Corrections, not the legislature.

The restorative justice movement is very dispersed in leadership and activity. It has many of the characteristics of a grassroots movement, although there is significant government involvement in some places. Without large amounts of money, high profile leadership or a marketing plan, the movement has, nevertheless, spread across the country in justice systems and is now influencing other fields such as education and social services. There is a remarkable level of coherence and focus in the movement, in spite of the lack of a national voice or organizing infrastructure.

For the most part practitioners have been at the forefront of this movement rather than academicians and theoreticians. It was Howard Zehr's direct experience in doing victim offender mediation that led to the theory he describes in *Changing Lenses* (1990), the foundational book of the current restorative justice movement.

Developments in the field have sometimes defied the expectations of restorative justice practitioners themselves. The early victim-offender mediation practitioners assumed that victim-offender mediation would never be used in cases of serious violent crime. However, several victims of serious crime, wanting something to help them move on in their lives, insisted on the opportunity to meet with the offender. Facilitating face-to-face meetings in cases of severe violence is now a growing area of practice and research with formal programs in at least nine states.

Restorative justice practices are generally appended to the mainstream system and supported by discretionary or soft money. To move past being a novelty for a few cases to become a normal way of doing business in the justice system, it will be necessary to shift resources more systemically and infuse all activities and functions of the justice system with restorative values.

WHAT ARE THE CHALLENGES FACING RESTORATIVE PRACTICE?

Balancing the Need for Flexibility and Responsivity and the Desire to Standardize

The process of creating restorative responses to crime is necessarily holistic, circular, shaped by those closest to the problem, responsive the specifics of the situation (not universal) and messy. At the same time there is a need to describe and quantify what is happening to be accountable to the larger society and ensure fairness and appropriateness.

Maintaining a Focus on Victims' Needs and Concerns

Very often victims are not involved or are brought into the planning and implementation of restorative practices as an afterthought. It takes great vigilance to avoid slipping into the habit of framing everything around offenders. For example, people often begin with the question, "For what kinds of offenses is restorative justice appropriate?" That question centers on the offender. What happens if we ask, "For what kinds of hurts is restorative justice appropriate?"

Staying True to the Values of the New Paradigm

Any new way of doing work faces a strong tendency for older, familiar patterns to reassert themselves. Over time key elements of practice may become blurred or erode. Time pressures, lack of a sense of competence in the new way, lack of training, resistance to change–all of these factors can cause practitioners to take short cuts or do it the old way.

Reducing Dependence on Professionals

Several decades of referring more and more community problems to professional services (e.g., police, social services) have eroded community skills and sense of efficacy in handling community problems. Many lay people do not speak up, or they defer to professional opinions, waiting for the experts to solve the problem. Professional skills and knowledge have an important contribution to make, but they are only one source of information and resources. Community insight, skills and resources can make a much greater contribution than is currently the case.

Using the Full Capacity of Restorative Processes

Many programs deal only with first time offenders and very low-level cases, which might be more readily resolved in an informal community or family process and should not enter the criminal justice system at all. Restorative processes have the capacity to deal with very difficult situations, and, because they are generally more time intensive, using them for primarily low-level offenses fails to take advantage of their full potential in improving community life.

Integrating Values into Technique

In restorative justice, how to be with people is as important as what to do with people. Actions are not independent of core values. Specific techniques, formulas for action, are subject to contextual determination and cannot be rigidly set. Yet as a culture we do not have much patience for discussions of values, neither do we give much thought to how we intentionally apply values on a daily basis to guide decisions within a span of options available. Criminal justice professionals frequently say, "Just tell me what to do." Action without understanding the underlying values can produce results contrary to the intention.

Sufficient Referrals

In many community-based programs, we find the paradox of unused community capacity to handle cases and an overloaded system. Even in jurisdictions sympathetic to restorative programs, it is a challenge to provide a steady flow of referrals. The habits and momentum of the system are difficult to modify to create a nonstandard channel for cases. Many programs whose services are primarily delivered by community volunteers find that they spend more time trying to get referrals than they do in maintaining their volunteer corps.

Creating a Workable Interface with an Adversarial System

Restorative processes build relationships and trust. Truth telling is considered essential to developing effective solutions. If a person who reveals information out of trust is then thrust into an adversarial process that threatens harm or feels very disrespectful, the person will understandably experience a sense of betrayal of the trust extended. Issues of confidentiality are very thorny in practice.

Openly Articulating a Commitment to Compassion and Love in Our Work

Ironically, love and compassion are thought of as soft, when in fact it takes much more courage to speak of love and compassion than to speak of hate and vengeance in public discourse. Compassion and our capacity to connect as human beings are at the core of restorative philosophy. Accountability is a natural by-product of healthy love. If we love someone, we know it does harm to his/her soul to harm others and that the way to heal the soul is to take responsibility and to make amends. Healthy love is the environment most conducive for a wrongdoer to take full responsibility and to make the changes necessary to make sure it won't happen again. Healthy love does not excuse behavior or run away from responsibility. Walking the path of compassion is extremely hard work–it's not for the faint of heart.

CONCLUSION

Restorative justice philosophy is energizing a wide range of activities across the United States toward a vision of wholeness for all those harmed by crime. These restorative practices attempt to involve victims, offenders and community members in a partnership with the justice system to repair the harm of crime and reweave the fabric of the community. This shift in focus of the justice process challenges communities and the justice system to continuously examine the underlying value structure of practice and evaluation to determine whether the work done and the questions asked are consistent with the vision of healing and strengthening individuals and communities.

Restorative practices are expanding within the justice system and in other fields. Significant challenges face practitioners as they craft responses to crime that share pain, seek a path of healing and move toward hope through inclusion, respect, shared decision-making and mutual responsibility. Research to date is promising, but incomplete. There is much to learn about how to most effectively achieve restorative outcomes.

The restorative justice movement is deeply rooted in values of interdependence and non-domination. Holding those values in healthy balance requires continuous dialog with deep listening. Honoring each individual as a unique and indispensable part of the larger whole supports people in acting on behalf of their own well-being in balance with the well-being of others. The task of restorative justice is to create spaces in which people can experience one another through heart and spirit and can access their own capacity for wisdom and healing through relationships with others.

A colleague from education, after listening to several people discuss restorative justice, said, "Oh, I get it. It's like 30 years ago when we threw a bottle out the window, we thought we threw it away. Then the environmental movement taught us: There is no "away." Wherever we throw it, it is still part of us. Restorative justice says the same about people." The restorative justice movement calls for mindfulness about our connections and our impact on one another. That is the basis for healthy living in our families, schools, neighborhoods, workplaces, and in the justice system.

REFERENCES

Achilles, M. & Zehr, H. (2001). Restorative Justice for Crime Victims: The Promise, the Challenge. In G. Bazemore & M. Schiff (Eds.), Restorative Community Justice: Repairing Harm and Transforming Communities. Cincinnati, OH: Anderson Publishing.

Bazemore, G. (2000). Rock and Roll, Restorative Justice, and the Continuum of the Real World: A Response to "Purism" in Operationalizing Restorative Justice. *Contemporary Justice Review*, 3(4), 459-477.

Bazemore, G. (2001). Young People, Trouble, and Crime: Restorative Justice as a Normative Theory of Informal Social Control and Social Support. *Youth and Society*, 33(2), 199-226.

Bazemore, B., Nissen, L., & Dooley, M. (2000). Mobilizing Social Support and Building Relationships: Broadening Correctional and Rehabilitative Agendas, unpublished paper.

Bazemore, G. & Schiff, M. (Eds.). (2001). Restorative and Community Justice: Repairing Harm and Transforming Communities. Cincinnati, OH: Anderson Publishing.

Braithwaite, J. (2001). Restorative Justice and Responsive Regulation. New York: Oxford University Press.

Braithwaite, J. & Petit, P. (1990). Not Just Desserts: A Republican Theory of Criminal Justice. Oxford, UK: Oxford University Press.

Coates, R., Umbreit, M., & Voss, B. (2000). Restorative Justice Circles in South Saint Paul, Minnesota. St. Paul, MN: Center for Restorative Justice and Peacemaking, University of Minnesota.

Couture, J., Parker, T., Couture, R., & Laboucane, P. (2001). A Cost-Benefit Analysis of Hollow Water's Community Holistic Healing Process. Ottawa, ON: Solicitor General of Canada.

Dalai Lama. (1999). Ethics for the New Millennium. New York, NY: Riverhead Books.

Hammond, S.A. (1996). The Thin Book of Appreciative Inquiry. Plano, TX: Thin Book Publishing Co.

Karp, D. & Breslin, B. (2001). Restorative Justice in School Communities. *Youth and Society*, 33(2), 249-272.

Kuhn, T. (1962). The Structure of Scientific Revolutions. Chicago, IL: University of Chicago Press.

Latimer, J., Dowden, C., & Muise, D. (2001). The Effectiveness of Restorative Justice Practices: A Meta-Analysis. Ottawa, ON: Department of Justice Canada.

Lofland, J. & Lofland, L. (1995). Analyzing Social Settings: A Guide to Qualitative Observation and Analysis (3rd Edition). London: Wadsworth Publishing Co.

Maloney, D., Bazemore, G., & Hudson, J. (2001). The End of Probation and the Beginning of Community corrections. *Perspectives* (Summer 2001): 23-30.

McCold, P. (2000). "Toward a Holistic Vision of Restorative Juvenile Justice: A Reply to the Minimalist Model. *Contemporary Justice Review*, 3(4): 357-372.

Miller, R.Y. (1996). Cloudhand, Clenched Fist: Chaos, Crisis, and the Emergence of Community. San Diego, CA: LuraMedia Inc.

Patton, M. (1990). Qualitative Evaluation and Research Methods (2nd Ed.). Newbury, CA: Sage Publications Inc.

Pranis, K. (1992). Incarceration vs. Rehabilitation vs. Restorative Justice. Unpublished paper presented in Rochester, MN, to Dodge-Fillmore-Ohmsted Community Corrections Advisory Board.

Pranis, K. (1994). Restorative Justice Asks These Questions. St. Paul, MN: MN Department of Corrections.

Pranis, K. (1997). Rethinking Community Corrections: Restorative Values and an Expanded Role for the Community. *The ICCA Journal on Community Corrections*, 8(1): 36-39.

Pranis, K. (2001). Restorative Justice, Social Justice, and the Empowerment of Marginalized Populations. In G. Bazemore & M. Schiff (Eds.), Restorative Community Justice: Repairing Harm and Transforming Communities. Cincinnati, OH: Anderson Publishing.

Roberts, T. (1995). Evaluation of the Victim Offender Mediation Project, Langely, BC: Final Report. Victoria, BC: Focus Consultants.

Umbreit, M. (1999). Avoiding the Marginalization and the McDonalization of Victim Offender Mediation: A Case Study in Moving Toward the Mainstream. In G. Bazemore & L. Walgrave (Eds.), Restorative Juvenile Justice: Repairing the Harm of Youth Crime. Monsey, NY: Criminal Justice Press.

Umbreit, M., Coates, R., & Voss, B. (2001). Victim Offender Mediation & Dialog in Crimes of Severe Violence. Retrieved November 20, 2002, from http://sww.che.umn.edu/rjp.

Umbreit, M., Coates, R., & Voss, B. (2002). The Impact of Restorative Justice Conferencing: A Review of 63 Empirical Studies in 5 Countries. Retrieved November 20, 2002, from http://sww.che.umn.edu/rjp.

Van Ness, D. & Strong, K.H. (2001). Restoring Justice (2nd Ed.). Cincinnati, OH: Anderson Publishing Co.

Walgrave, L. (2000). How Pure Can a Maximalist Approach to Restorative Justice Remain? Or Can a Purist Model of Restorative Justice Become Maximalist? *Contemporary Justice Review*, 3(4): 415-432.

Zehr, H. (1990). Changing Lenses: A New Focus for Crime and Justice. Scottsdale, PA: Herald Press.

Zehr, H. (2002). The Little Book of Restorative Justice. Intercourse, PA: Good Books.

From Fury to Forgiveness

Marietta Jaeger Lane

SUMMARY. This autobiographical piece chronicles the kidnap and subsequent murder of the author's youngest daughter during a camping vacation in Montana and the author's spiritual journey from hate to healing. Once the case was resolved, Jaeger Lane relates the impact of this event as a speaking/writing ministry evolved around the issues of forgiveness, reconciliation and advocating for the abolition of the death penalty as a person of faith and as the mother of a murder victim. She ends with her experience of seeing first-hand the success of utilizing restorative justice principles in the rehabilitation of errants and addicts. *Article copies available for a fee from The Haworth Document Delivery Service: 1-800-HAWORTH. E-mail address: <docdelivery@haworth press.com> Website: <http://www.HaworthPress.com> © 2004 by The Haworth Press, Inc. All rights reserved.]*

KEYWORDS. Victim, forgiveness, justice, death penalty, healing, lifers

"Mama! There's a hole in the tent and Susie's gone!" Those words, cried out in panic by my oldest daughter, Heidi, slashed into my sleep

Marietta Jaeger Lane is a Founding Board Member of Murder Victims Families For Reconciliation (MVFR) and Journey of Hope . . . From Violence to Healing, national organizations led by and comprised primarily of murder victim family members who oppose the death penalty. Her story has been documented in many media; she is an international speaker, has been interviewed by The Vatican Radio and testified before the United Nations Commission on Human Rights in Geneva, Switzerland.

[Haworth co-indexing entry note]: "From Fury to Forgiveness." Lane, Marietta Jaeger. Co-published simultaneously in *Journal of Religion & Spirituality in Social Work* (The Haworth Social Work PraticePress, an imprint of The Haworth Press, Inc.) Vol. 23, No. 1/2, 2004, pp. 159-172; and: *Criminal Justice: Retribution vs. Restoration* (ed: Eleanor Hannon Judah, and Rev. Michael Bryant) The Haworth Social Work Practice Press, an imprint of The Haworth Press, Inc., 2004, pp. 159-172. Single or multiple copies of this article are available for a fee from The Haworth Document Delivery Service [1-800-HAWORTH, 9:00 a.m. - 5:00 p.m. (EST). E-mail address: docdelivery@haworthpress.com].

and exposed me to the worst nightmare of my life. It was the middle of the night and my parents, husband and our five children were camped at the Missouri River Headwaters State Park in southwestern Montana. We'd arrived only three days before, at this our first stop on a month-long camping vacation through this beautiful mountainous state. Our plan had been to depart for the next campground on our itinerary in the morning. But now, suddenly, Susie was gone–my precious precocious seven-year-old youngest–stolen from her family through a hole in our tent, cut under cover of the midnight sky!

We grabbed flashlights, frantically running around the campground in a futile attempt to find her. My husband and dad drove into the closest town of Three Forks to alert the town Marshall, who, after notifying the county Sheriff and the FBI, arrived quickly on the scene. As dawn broke and campers awoke, some readying for an early departure, law enforcement officials searched tents, trailers and vehicles before anyone was allowed to leave. Deputies conducted a wide-ranging search of all buildings. Military men came with tracking dogs, search-and-rescue teams scoured the area for miles around, and ranchers checked every crevice of the farthest reaches of their lands–all in search of Susie.

Several days later, a mysterious garbled call about the kidnapping came to an FBI office in another state, thus enabling the FBI to take charge of the investigation. A camper was installed near us as "headquarters." Suspects were questioned and given lie-detector tests; sightings of children and clues were checked out, hundreds of persons joined in the search throughout the state. All we could do was stay at our campsite to watch and wonder, hope and pray, and wait.

A week after Susie's disappearance, a call came to the home of a deputy working on the case, identifying Susie by an unpublished birth defect and asking a large sum of money for ransom. Although the message lacked all the details need to carry out the ransom exchange, we prepared as much as possible. Not hearing again from the kidnapper after a week, we held a press conference at the campground, appealing to him through the media for another contact with final arrangements. No word was forthcoming. Meanwhile, myriad investigative activities and searches continued to take place all around us and well beyond. Still, all we could do was watch, pray, and wait some more.

Finally, came the day which pushed me over the edge, but eventually and fortunately, into the arms of God. Throughout the day, search planes droned overhead, waving to us as they circled the campground and then flying off to another fruitless search. All day long, police boats dragged the river beside us, and every time the boat stopped to examine the contents of their nets, my heart stopped too. All day long, I saw the toll of this terrible experience in my other four children. I could not bear to look into my husband's face, to see his anguish that he could not save his youngest daughter. I imaged what I would do if the kidnapper were standing before me. In the intensity and exhaustion of that harrowing day, my concern and fears for my daughter gave way to roiling anger, searing hatred, and a vicious desire for the torturous death of this person who had caused this to happen.

That night as I crawled into bed, I confessed to my husband, "Even if the kidnapper were to bring Susie back this moment, alive and well, I could kill him for what he has done to our family!" I meant it with every fiber of my being and I knew I could do it, with my bare hands and a big smile on my face. However, I no sooner turned over to sleep, when I heard very clearly, "But that's not how I want you to feel." Well, I knew that Christians are called to forgive their enemies, but this was different–Susie was an innocent, defenseless child and I was her mother. It was right and proper for me to avenge anything terrible that happened to her. And, at that time in Montana, the penalty for kidnapping was the death penalty–I wanted this guy to swing!

"But that's not how I want you to feel." I recognized that God was asking me to let go of my rage and desire for revenge, but I felt absolutely justified and everyone around me would support me in that stance. I knew I'd be allowed to give input about the kidnapper's sentence when he was caught and I wanted him to pay and pay plenty! He deserved all the punishment he could get! "But that's not how I want you to feel." God was calling me to let go of my hate–the violence within *me*–and I was resisting, refusing, justified and righteous, so very human. Through long night hours, I argued my case, I wrestled with God.

God had prepared me for this moment; I knew the principles to which I would be accountable if I was to live my life with integrity as a Catholic Christian. And even in purely psychological terms, I knew that hatred was not healthy. I'd seen for myself, in family members and friends, the unhappiness and unhealthiness that anger and unforgiveness brings. I also knew myself well enough to know that I was an all-or-nothing kind of person–if I gave myself to that kind of rage and revenge, it would obsess and consume me and, in the end, I'd be no good or help for anyone. I realized that what God was asking me to do was the best I could do for myself, for Susie and for my family. I also know now that there were many people praying for me when I could not, holding me before the face of God, so that I could say "yes" to God when I should. God is faithful. In the middle of the night, I surrendered.

However, that is not to say that I immediately forgave the kidnapper. I could not deny the adverse feelings still in my heart. What I *was* able to do was to *give God permission to change my heart,* because I believe in a God who never violates the gift of our free will, and I promised to co-operate with whatever my Creator could do to heal me and move my heart from fury to forgiveness. At that point also, I committed myself to be as faithful to Susie as I believe God to me, that is to keep searching for her, believing her to be alive, until such time, if it ever had to happen, that I had to accept concrete proof to the contrary. With those prayers, though I still had no answers about my little girl, I felt a huge burden lift from me and was able to sleep well the rest of the night. Several weeks later, we had to return to our home in Michigan, still without Susie.

Three months later, the kidnapper called—a brief call answered by my oldest son, in which Susie was again correctly identified by an unpublished birth defect. He declared his intention was still to return her for ransom but hadn't yet devised a plan to do so. He said he'd call when that happened. Once again, all we could do was hope, pray, wait and wait and wait.

The fall and winter holidays passed, not knowing what kind of a holiday Susie was having. Then came months and months of an emotional roller-coaster ride—having our hopes raised and then dashed as more suspects were questioned and then released, reports of other children thought to be Susie were resolved and clues determined to be irrelevant to our case.

Finally, it became almost a year since the kidnapping; the Montana press wanted to print an interview about what it was like to endure that long a time without knowing how my little girl was, where she was, even *if* she was, anymore. By mistake, the article was printed the day before the actual first year anniversary date, but by the providence of God, included a verbatim statement in which I was quoted, "I'd give anything to talk to the kidnapper myself, but after all this time having elapsed, I doubt it is possible."

The kidnapper read that article, was challenged by my statement, and the following night, in the middle of the night, *one year to the minute* that he'd taken Susie out of our tent, called me at our home in Michigan. The call woke me from a sound sleep but answering the phone, I instantly knew who the caller was. Identifying Susie by her unpublished birth defect to prove his authenticity, he said he still wanted to exchange her for ransom but still had not yet devised a plan to do so where he would not be caught. Mostly, it soon became apparent that he really had called just to taunt me. "You wanted to talk to me. Here I am. What good is it going to do for you? I am the one who is in control. Nothing will happen until *I* say it will."

But something very remarkable had happened *to me* as I first heard his voice on the phone. From that time a year ago in Montana when I had chosen to say "yes" to God and work toward an attitude of forgiveness, I had tried to be faithful to my promise. Daily, I prayed and read Scripture. Daily, sometimes even hourly, I reminded myself that, however *I* felt about the kidnapper, *in God's eyes this person was as precious to God as my little girl*. That is the kind of God I say I believe in—a God who is crazy about each and every one of us, no matter who we are and whatever we may have done—and so, in essence, I had to put my money where my faith was. Even if this man was not behaving like a Son of God, he *was* a Son of God, a member of God's family, and as such he had dignity and worth, as we all do—not by any merit of our own but because Jesus died for God and us has chosen to love us all. Pragmatically, that meant that I had to think and speak of the kidnapper with respectful terms and not use the derogatory ones that others used and which came so easily to my mind, given that for months I'd not known what Susie had to endure. I had to exercise self-control, "sit on my tongue" and be very careful about the language I used in reference to the kidnapper. I also knew that, as a Christian, I was to pray for my enemies.

Certainly this man fit that category, but in the beginning that was the last thing I felt like doing—I wanted him to be as miserable as we all were! However, my parents and the good nuns who educated me had deeply instilled the virtue of obedience, and so, if for no other reason, I attempted to comply.

At first, the best I could muster was to give an assent, so to speak, to God blessing him just once a day. My prayers were simple and unsophisticated; I had no idea who this person was and what his lifestyle. So I'd pray that if he was travelling, may he not have car trouble or that the weather would be right for his activities or if he was hunting or fishing, may he have a good catch. But I discovered one of God's holy tricks—when we pray for someone else to change, our own heart becomes changed. The more I prayed for this man, the more *I* realized how much he needed God's love and blessing in his life; certainly, if he still had Susie, I wanted him to be good to her; if he didn't have her any longer, I wanted him to have the courage to confess what had happened. Only if this person knew God and experiencing God's blessing and providence loved him could any of this be realized. My prayers became more frequent and fervent.

I will never pretend or claim that forgiveness is easy. Forgiveness is hard work. It takes daily diligent discipline. It takes prayer and fasting. It is counter to the way of the world, our own humanness and the work of the powers and principalities. Because we are human, we need time and space to process *all* our feelings and heal to forgiveness. When we do forgive, we are not condoning the act that has been done–I will never say that kidnapping my daughter is okay with me! Forgiveness is not forgetting–in fact it is precisely because we can*not ever forget* what has been done, that we *must* learn to forgive, so that we will not remain enslaved to a past event *that can never, ever be undone*, and *will be our own undoing* unless we can move on with our lives in a healthy, caring and peaceful manner. Forgiveness is the only way we can set ourselves free to do so.

God knows how each of us has suffered, that we're left weak and helpless in our loss, pain and anguish, but we also need to remember that God loves us too much to give us principles and commandments to live by and leave us powerless to do so. That's why God gives us a share in the life of Jesus–the Holy Spirit. That Life of Jesus comes to us at a dear and precious price, the death of God's own beloved Son–*the Son whom God cherished*–and God does not want to waste a single moment of Jesus' suffering. That power is, and will be, always available–however we need it, whenever we ask for it. The Holy Spirit, received at Baptism, living in us, and our own co-creative/cooperative work with God, are the means by which our hearts are changed and we become fully capable of mercy, compassion and forgiveness, with no strings attached. These are the truths that I came to realize, stumbling and bumbling in the process as I did, during that long year of waiting.

So finally, now, on the first anniversary of that year, standing in my kitchen in my nightgown in the middle of the night, one year to the minute that the kidnapper had taken my little girl from me, I was talking to the man who did so. Even though he was being smug and nasty, as I listened to his voice, I knew that all I'd been working and praying for, in terms of moving my heart from fury to forgiveness, had come to fruition in me. No longer was it a matter of intellect or will; now it was truly a "done-deed" in my heart. And, it made all the difference as to what happened next.

This man had called with the intent of taunting, frustrating and infuriating me, hoping to hear me hysterical, getting his kicks and then hanging up, letting me hang on for months again. Instead, what happened was that he was utterly undone by what God had done in me. He stayed on the phone for over an hour, *even though it was obvious* that the call was being traced, with all kinds of clicks easily heard on the line. He said he'd come to love Susie as his own daughter; he answered many of my questions truthfully because he did not expect to be caught. Then, when I said I'd been praying for him and asked what I could do for him, there was a long silence. Very softly at first, I began to hear him crying. "I wish this burden could be taken from me," he sobbed, and though I knew the possibilities of what that "burden" could be, I could not get him to elaborate. All I could hope for was that he *had* felt the love of God and had been deeply touched. The call ended and I was left listening to the dial tone.

The telephone trace failed. I thought my heart would break because he'd said that Susie was "right up the hill in my cabin" and I so longed to know it was truly so. However–a sign that God was still at work–I had remembered to turn on the recorder attached to the phone before I picked up the receiver; the whole call was on tape. When the FBI agents in Montana listened to it, they found that, in the conversation's milieu of concern and compassion, the kidnapper had let down his guard and inadvertently revealed enough information that they were able to identify him–a local man, David.

When David was told he was now considered the prime suspect in Susie's disappearance, on his attorney's advice, he took a lie detector test and then, a truth serum test, in a carefully monitored hospital situation to insure protection of all his rights. He "passed" them both! But on the way home from the hospital that night, he attempted to abduct another young girl on a Girl Scout campout. I praise God that the children woke up, the intruder frightened away and the abduction foiled, but all evidence pointed to David as the perpetrator.

Now it became evident that the FBI had to safeguard the community from a very sick man and a grave danger to children but without being able to arrest him. They had to wait for a not-yet-available expert witness who could ensure a successful prosecution, which would disallow David's release and return into the community to do more harm. In an effort to precipitate a resolution, they asked me to come back to Montana to confront David face-to-face, in the hopes that, as he'd broken down on the anniversary phone call, he would again break down in my presence.

I was grateful for this God-given opportunity–to say to David, face-to-face and not just to a voice on the phone, that I had forgiven him and that God was giving him this opportunity to receive the help he so desperately needed. But David and his attorney had to agree to my coming, and David had ample time to be on guard, be in good control of himself and was very careful not to incriminate himself in any way. After three fruitless encounters, I had to give it all back to God and the FBI, and returned to Michigan.

Something, however, in our conversations had piqued David, and a week later he eluded surveillance, drove all night long in another man's truck to Salt Lake City, Utah, where he called me "collect," so it could easily be traced, the next morning. His attempted ruse was to convince the FBI and me that the *real* kidnapper was someone else in Salt Lake City, not the prime suspect, David, in Montana. I recognized David's voice, knew he was the one who had taken Susie but kept asking questions to keep him on the line, aware the call was being traced. As we talked, I began to call him David, which he protested: "I'm not David. David is the man in Montana who the FBI think took Susie, but he's really innocent. I'm the one who has her." I continued to call him by name till he panicked and became confused and frantic, rehashing our conversations of the week before in Montana, which had been witnessed by his own attorney and FBI agents. He had already identified Susie by her unpublished birth defect, and now he was totally incriminating *himself*. When he realized this, he snarled, "You'll never see your little girl again," and slammed down the phone and sped away. Once again, I was left listening only to the dial tone.

But, I had taped this call with David's unintended admission of guilt and it was what the FBI needed to finally seek a warrant. Everything in readiness, the Agent-in-Charge, by now a dear friend, called to inform me of David's impending arrest, asking me not to discuss the case with the media, as I was to be a primary witness in the trial. However, he also had to tell me that nine months after Susie's disappearance, an eighteen-year-old girl had also disappeared from the town in which both she and David lived, her remains were found two weeks later on an abandoned ranch up in the hills beyond the campground. David had been an original suspect in *her* death, but he'd been excused after passing a lie detector test. Now, however, that a connection had also been made between David and Susie, they'd gone back to the abandoned ranch, taken it apart with shovel and back-hoe, and sent all their findings to the Smithsonian Institute in Washington, DC to be examined by anthropologists and biologists. That very day the FBI received a report that the last bundle had contained part of a *little* girl's backbone.

It was the concrete proof of what I had already come to know in my heart–that even though David talked about exchanging Susie for ransom, her life had been taken from her about a week after she'd been taken from us. All this time we'd been searching for her, she was already safely home, in the arms of God–not the answer I'd been praying for–but God was faithful to comfort and help me through that grief-filled and desolate night, and there were many people praying for me.

The next morning, David was arrested, still protesting his innocence. After he was incarcerated, the FBI, with warrants in hand, searched his home and therein found irrefutable evidence as to his guilt. David's attorney, who had heretofore genuinely believed in his client's innocence, returned to the jail with the agents and deputies. It was time for "justice" to be done.

In the last intervening fifteen months since Susie had been taken, I had spent much time praying and studying Scripture, trying to understand what genuine "justice" was. Now I was convinced that *God's idea of justice was not punishment but restoration.* In the simplest terms, as a Catholic Christian, I believe that Jesus is the "Word" of God made Flesh. Therefore, Jesus has to be the "Justice" of God made Flesh.

When I studied the life of Jesus in Scripture, I did not see someone who came to punish and destroy us, hurt us or put us to death. I did see someone who came to heal and help us, rehabilitate and reconcile us, and *restore to us* the life that Scripture says was lost to us by the sin of Adam and Eve. From all of Scripture, both the Hebrew and Christian books, rose up a God of mercy and compassion, who forgave us over and over again, who longed to share the glories of eternity with all of us forever–so much so that that God sent Jesus to live his life and give his life, so that *we could be restored* to the life for which God had really created us.

I did not know if David could ever be "restored"–he was a very sick young man–but I did not want to deny him the opportunity God wants for all of us–of repentance, rehabilitation, and restitution. However, the usual sentence for kidnap/murder in Montana was the death penalty, something to which heretofore I'd never given much thought, having lived all my life in Michigan, which has never had capital punishment. I struggled with this issue. I knew that forgiveness did not mean absolving of responsibility. For his own good and growth, David needed to be held accountable to the degree appropriate to his serious mental illness. That would be part of the restorative nature of justice.

In Montana, his accountability meant execution. Neither could I advocate forgiving violent persons and putting them back on the street; I know too well the cost of that violence. What I really wanted was for the violence and killing to stop and I realized that that included in the prison death chamber too. As I said before, I am an all-or-nothing person and that meant either all life is sacred or none of it is. As a Catholic Christian, the former was the value and guide I chose. What also concerned me was how I could best honor my daughter's precious memory. I felt that to kill someone in her name would profane and violate the sweetness, innocence and loveliness of her life. Susie was worthy of a more beautiful, honorable and noble memorial than a cold-blooded, pre-meditated, state-sanctioned killing of a chained, defenseless person, however deserving of death one may deem him to be. I knew I would better honor her memory by aspiring to a higher moral principle, befitting the goodness of her life; one that proclaimed *all of life* was worthy of preservation. Now, I knew I had to oppose the imposition of the death penalty.

The FBI and the County Prosecutor understood by then that it was my wish that the only alternative sentence be given, a mandatory life sentence with no chance of parole, but with the opportunity for psychiatric help. They, happily of the same mindset, honored my hopes and allowed David's attorney to bargain for that opportunity in exchange for a full confession. Only then was David willing to confess to four deaths committed in that county—Susie's, the young woman's and two young boys'—in separate situations several years before Susie's death. I was to hear that there was nothing I could think of that didn't happen to my little girl in the week or so she was held captive, either before her death or after. Then, to compound my horror and grief, David hung himself in his jail cell four hours after his confession.

That was not what I'd wanted, hoped and prayed for, for David, but I had to accept his death as I'd had to accept Susie's, in faith and trust that God would bring good and life from all these terrible events, as God had done from the death of Jesus.

Finally we had all our answers and a month later, the FBI quietly slipped my husband and I back into Montana, where we buried her few remains. After the simple funeral, I went to visit David's mother. Her experience of him was of a devoted, respectful, loving son. I couldn't imagine how she was dealing with this heretofore-unknown facet of his personality and all the horrible things he'd done to children. I hoped it would help her, a committed Christian and innocent victim, to know I'd forgiven David. Though still stunned, numb and reeling, she received me graciously and together we were able to hold each other and grieve the loss of our children. Since then, we have prayed often with each other at Susie and David's graves.

Through the years, faithful as God always is, many good and life-giving things have come from these tragic deaths. I am so grateful for God's persistence in challenging and teaching me to forgive, as I was the first recipient of God's blessing. I know I am much happier and healthier now than had I stayed with my rage. Twenty-seven years of working with other murder victim family members has affirmed and confirmed my own experience. They all have a valid right to the normal, initial human response of anger, hatred and even a desire for revenge, but those who *continue* to retain a vindictive mindset, however justified they feel, only give the offender another victim–themselves. They hold onto their hate because they believe it gives them some control in a situation where they had no control, but in truth they have given control of their emotions and lives over to the person who is the cause of their pain! They become embittered and unhappy; the quality of their lives, their health and their relationships diminish.

More and more, the medical profession is discovering that often the root causes of our mental and physical problems, also our addictions, are hatred, resentment and unforgiveness. Unless we are willing to admit our angry feelings and process them in a helpful, healthy way, they will eventually manifest themselves on other levels of our being in a deleterious way. It's no wonder that forgiveness is a primary tenet in the world's major religions; God wants to heal us all and God knows the only way we can grow to be healthy, happy and holy people is when we learn to forgive.

A very special blessing that also happened is the founding of two national life-giving organizations, Murder Victims Families For Reconciliation (MVFR) and Journey of Hope . . . From Violence to Healing. Both these sister organizations are comprised primarily of people like me, people who have lost a loved one to murder, including families of the executed. Naturally, all initially were filled with deep grief and rage, but eventually came to the realization that the only way they could heal, properly honor the memories of their loved ones lost to violence, and live out their lives in a healthy manner was to let go of their hate and move to forgiveness and reconciliation.

The members of both groups are opposed to the death penalty; our cry is "Don't kill in our names!" We know that we cannot honor the lives of our beloved dead by becoming that which we abhor–people who kill people. We know that executions only make more victims and more grieving families. Many are involved in prison ministries, campaigning for just trials and prison reform, or are working to save inmates, sometimes the offender in their own case, from death row. All of us are willing to share our painfully personal, incredibly varied, stories of violence and victims, from hate to healing as we are invited, and also on speaking tours organized by local activists throughout states that are killing prisoners.

Though every one of us would give all we have *not to be able to speak* with credibility and authority about the murder of family members and the death penalty, God has blessed our efforts by making our presentations powerful and persuasive arguments against capital punishment. No one can say to us, "Well, if it happened to your loved one, you wouldn't be opposed to the death penalty." It did and we are.

Almost from the beginning, without any intent or design on my part, God seemed to orchestrate the evolvement of a speaking ministry about forgiveness, based on my own struggle and education, which has, amazingly, through the years, taken me around the world! More importantly, as people have listened, God has spoken through Susie's story and helped them to recognize areas in their own lives where a spirit of unforgiveness has kidnapped them from the safety of God's tent. Hearing how God helped me in such a situation gives them the courage to call on God for help for themselves.

I have been blessed many times to be invited to give presentations to, and visit with, inmates in prisons and penitentiaries across our country and Canada. What I have heard from them, again and again, is the desire to be forgiven by their victims as a means to their own healing and their own need to forgive those whose terrible treatment of them set the stage for their own violent behavior, for which they now sit in their cold, hard, steel and cement cells. However, most often, communication from inmates to victims/victims' families is disallowed by the legal system, and the punitive measures mandated by law or practiced as policy or in secret by prison personnel only continue to reinforce violent behaviors. Educations, rehabilitation, healing of hurting and disabled human beings are not a concern in most facilities. And therefore, many are lost in despair, desolation and destruction. A tragic waste of life!

The media and the politicians incite and promote the fears and anger of our communities and so we agree to provide tax dollars for more punitive legislation and brutal prisons. Yet, most inmates will complete their sentences and return to our neighborhoods. I wonder when people scream for the authorities to "get tough on crime," who they'd want living next door to them–an ex-inmate who's become literate, goes to AA meetings, been given job training and affirmed as a worthwhile person, who has developed nonviolent conflict resolution skills or a person who's been kept locked up in near-isolation, brutalized, dehumanized and comes out meaner and angrier than before!

The truth is that we are all more than our worst action; there is the capacity for goodness, creativity and love in everyone, even those who have committed the most heinous crime. I can never bring myself to even imagine what Susie had to endure, yet David, as mentally ill as he was, took good care of his mother, was a competent and industrious worker, had a perfect four-year record while in the Marines and was a well-liked, good friend to those who knew him. On the anniversary call, he was capable of tears of remorse when he experienced God loving him through me. When he was arrested, though many people were not surprised, just as many would not believe he was guilty. David was as capable of doing good as he was of evil behavior.

We must find a way to utilize our money, resources, laws, people-power, educational systems and facilities to develop programs that bring out the best in our incarcerated offenders, programs which develop intellectual growth, latent talents and abilities, programs that heal, humanize and offer hope. I'm certain other entries in this volume will propose just such programs, activities and legislation.

One area that I've been privileged to partake of in prisons is faith-based gatherings–studies, liturgies and charitable services. As a woman whose own healing of a horrendous act of violence was centered on my relationship with God, the example of Jesus my brother and the power of the Holy Spirit, I admit my partiality to the rehabilitative power of authentic faith-based programs. Many times I have been honored to participate in worship services with lifers in prison. These men wake up to the same dismal scene and scenario every day of their lives; they live hourly with the knowledge that they have committed a terrible crime which, however their admission of total responsibility and deep remorse, can *never* be undone. Yet, amazingly, these men come to prayer, to worship, with genuine joy, praise and trust that God is with them! They are peacemakers in the yard, mentors in classrooms, mediators on the job and prayer-intercessors for their brother inmates–and their victims–in their cells. I am always deeply moved by their witness. To be with them is to be on sacred ground.

While it is very true that occasionally there are staff and guards who are able to see the potential for good in some inmates and are willing to promote the possibility for that, more often there is no one nor nothing in the prison system which nurtures the inmates' development as caring, respectful, responsible human beings.

Ideally, if no one else, it should be a chaplain, who is always there for them and believes in them, provides them with the means to know and grow–not in religiosity, but spiritually, humanly–and values *their* wisdom and insights. I think it's a moot question how the healing happens–through the direct compassion and grace of God or the person of God who lets God love the inmates through him/her and their ministry. I have often witnessed that eventual healing, redemption, rehabilitation and resurrection does indeed happen in the context of faith-based gatherings held in prison.

I have also seen heroic and successful programs initiated by the inmates themselves–heroic because they have to regularly struggle to surmount system-placed obstacles and constantly battle for the right, permissions and opportunities to carry out the work; successful because the programs have emanated from within their own midst, giving a credibility, attraction and trustworthiness an outside program may not have.

Often, the men have to write their own materials for "classroom" study; these may be exercises in resolving conflicts in prison in a nonviolent manner or simple moral questions relevant to their situations. Other times, the effort takes the form of a newsletter promoting good and healthy values, soliciting helpful and inspirational articles from other inmates, even from other prisons. Some of these papers enjoy a countrywide network of subscriptions and submissions. I have read quite a few and they are quality pieces, reflecting intelligence, wisdom and goodness, and pertinent to us all.

For many years, I gave presentations on forgiveness and reconciliation at a rehabilitation program for Catholic clergy beset by the addictions of alcohol and drugs. I would tell them jokingly that they were my favorite audience because they had fallen off their "pedestals." But their gift in this situation was the experience of their human frailties and knowing their own neediness for God's mercy and grace. Now, they can be much more effective and compassionate shepherds for the rest of us who wrestle daily with our own weaknesses and failings. So, too, has it been with the many good people I've met in prisons. They are marvelously effective in demonstrating, by the witness of their rehabilitated lives, confined though they are by concrete, steel and barbed wire, that God will never fail nor forsake us because God is crazy about each and every one of us, no matter who we are and what we've ever done. God is just; God is always faithful to forgive and restore all those who desire a new Life. Shouldn't we, the people of God, do likewise?

Building from the Ground Up:
Strategies for Creating
Safe and Just Communities

Jeremy Travis

SUMMARY. In an era of low crime rates and high imprisonment rates, the role of communities in producing safety and justice is open for critical reexamination. This article suggests that community resiliency is an unexplored factor in the recent drop in violent crime rates, and that community capacity is adversely affected by imprisonment policies, creating critical questions about the ability of community organizations to engage in partnerships on crime and justice topics. Drawing lessons from several community policing experiments, this article outlines a possible role for community engagement in reducing the current reliance on incarceration as a response to crime. *[Article copies available for a fee from The Haworth Document Delivery Service: 1-800-HAWORTH. E-mail address: <docdelivery@haworthpress.com> Website: <http://www.HaworthPress.com> © 2004 by The Haworth Press, Inc. All rights reserved.]*

Jeremy Travis, JD, MPA, is Senior Fellow, Justice Policy Center, Urban Institute, Washington, DC.

Address correspondence to: Jeremy Travis, The Urban Institute, Justice Policy Center, 2100 M Street, NW, Washington, DC 20037 (E-mail: jtravis@ui. urban.org).

The author would like to express his appreciation for research support from Louise Dyer and Meagan Funches.

The views expressed in this article are those of the author, and should not be attributed to the Urban Institute, their trustees, or their funders.

[Haworth co-indexing entry note]: "Building from the Ground Up: Strategies for Creating Safe and Just Communities." Travis, Jeremy. Co-published simultaneously in *Journal of Religion & Spirituality in Social Work* (The Haworth Social Work Practice Press, an imprint of The Haworth Press, Inc.) Vol. 23, No. 1/2, 2004, pp. 173-195; and: *Criminal Justice: Retribution vs. Restoration* (ed: Eleanor Hannon Judah, and Rev. Michael Bryant) The Haworth Social Work Practice Press, an imprint of The Haworth Press, Inc., 2004, pp. 173-195. Single or multiple copies of this article are available for a fee from The Haworth Document Delivery Service [1-800-HAWORTH, 9:00 a.m. - 5:00 p.m. (EST). E-mail address: docdelivery@haworthpress.com].

KEYWORDS. Community, policing, incarceration, prisoner reentry, community safety, crime

As we survey the American landscape of criminal justice policy in the first years of the new century, we face two remarkable facts. First, crime rates are at the lowest level in a generation. Second, imprisonment rates are at the highest level in a generation. Who would have thought, a decade ago at the height of the crack epidemic, that rates of violence would reach their lowest levels since the first victimization survey was conducted in the early 1970s (National Crime Victimization Survey, 1973)? Who would have thought, when the prison population started to grow in the early 1970s, that we would increase the per capita incarceration rate more than fourfold over the next quarter century? These facts define the new reality of crime and punishment in America.

Researchers and policy analysts are engaged in important debates about the causes for the decline in crime rates in America. An equally vigorous debate is underway about the impact of the nation's experiment in the expanded use of imprisonment. Recently, these debates have taken on new dimensions. As the crime decline has leveled off, we ask: What policies will keep crime rates low? As the prison population stabilizes with the end of the prison-building boom, we ask: What policies can reduce the national incarceration rate?

This article examines the possible role for community organizations in providing part of the answers to those new questions. The following sections argue that strong communities are indeed necessary ingredients in the development of policies that are designed to achieve the social goal of a safe and just society. Specifically, the chapter proposes that communities become active partners in the development and implementation of policies that keep crime rates low, reduce the use of prisons as a response to crime, and enhance the quality of justice overall.

This argument must face, however, the conundrum of community capacity. We have a strong research basis for the conclusion that communities played an important role in bringing about the crime reductions that have astounded the world and confounded the dire predictions of many experts. Yet, we can also hypothesize with a weaker research base that the nation's reliance on incarceration as a response to crime has diminished the capacity of communities to provide for their own safety. More ironic, the fourfold increase in incarceration rates has also undermined the ability of communities to perform the important work of providing for the safety of their occupants and reintegrating record numbers of ex-offenders.

This conundrum poses a unique challenge to those interested in building strong communities. It poses a parallel challenge to those interested in reducing crime and the reliance on imprisonment. Can these two distinct policy and advocacy sectors find common ground? This chapter addresses these questions by reviewing the recent history of the crime drop, with particular emphasis on the role of communities and the lessons from community policing innovations, and then reviews the impact of incarceration policies, with special focus on the community level effects. The concluding section discusses a potential role for community organizations in shifting the framework for criminal justice policies in America.

LESSONS FROM THE RISE AND FALL OF VIOLENCE IN AMERICA

With the onset of the crack cocaine epidemic in the mid-1980s, rates of violence, particularly gun-related violence by young people, started to rise sharply. Long established patterns of criminal behavior and arrest activity lost their hold. As Figure 1 shows, from 1976 to 1985, there had been a relatively stable pattern in arrest rates. Young people between the ages of 18 and 24 had the highest arrest rates, followed by adults between the ages of 25 and 34, and juveniles under the age of 18. But beginning in the mid-1980s, the patterns came unraveled. In less than a decade, arrest rates for violent crimes increased by 50 percent for the two older groups, rose by 70 percent for juveniles, and changed not at all for adults over age 35.

Not only was this increase in violence concentrated in young people, guns played an important role. Figure 2, which tracks arrests for homicide, tells the tale of guns and kids in the era of the crack epidemic. Between 1985 and 1993, the rate of arrest of juveniles (under age 18) for homicides with a gun more than quadrupled. For the 18- to 24-year-age group, the arrest rate for gun homicides tripled. For both age groups, arrests for homicides not involving guns remained stable (Blumstein, 1995).

These steep increases in key indicators in youth crime over the space of a few years were an unprecedented phenomenon. Politicians responded with calls for stricter sentencing, more police, more prisons,

FIGURE 1. Violent Crime Index Arrest Rates by Age, 1976-2000

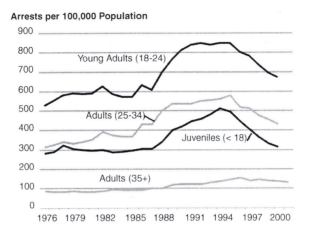

Source: Butts, J., and J. Travis. 2002. *The Rise and Fall of American Youth Violence: 1980 to 2000.* Washington, DC: The Urban Institute.

FIGURE 2. Gun and Non Gun Homicide Arrest Rates by Age, 1976-1999

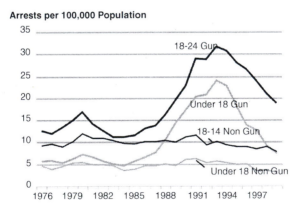

Source: Urban Institute Analysis of Data from Federal Bureau of Investigation, Supplementary Homicide Reports.

and more arrests. Some crime experts claimed that there was a new type of young criminal called a "superpredator." There were warnings that we should expect a "bloodbath of violence." For a few scary years, it indeed looked like youth violence in America's cities was spiraling out of control.

Looking back, we now know that these predictions were wrong. There was no bloodbath. Superpredators did not overrun our inner cities. The crack epidemic, which had prompted calls for stricter punishment and more stringent law enforcement, peaked in the early nineties. Street drug markets moved indoors. Young people started turning away from drug use, gun violence, and other risky behaviors. Beginning in 1992 rates of violent crime in America started to drop, then began to drop dramatically. By the turn of the century, according to the National Crime Victimization Survey, violence in America had reached the lowest levels since 1972 when the victim survey was first conducted.[1]

There has been a vigorous debate about the cause of the drop in crime rates. Some commentators credit new policing strategies, including the movement toward community policing, the adoption of "zero tolerance" policies, or the introduction of crime tracking technologies, such as the Compstat program in New York City (Eck & McGuire, 2000). Others point to the increase in incarceration in America and claim that the incapacitation of large numbers of individuals engaged in criminal behavior has reduced crime in our communities. Advocates of gun control policies point to federal restrictions on gun access, more aggressive enforcement of laws against gun trafficking, and the closing of thousands of federally licensed gun dealers as policies that have kept guns out of the hands of criminals. The strong economy of the 1990s is given credit for providing job opportunities for at risk young people. Some analysts point to shifting demographic patterns, suggesting that a decline in the number of young people in the crime producing years of life has provided a beneficial reduction in criminal activity.

There is some truth to all of these hypotheses (Blumstein & Wallman, 2000). Yet two possible contributors to the decline in crime in America, both relevant to the discussion in this article, have received little scholarly attention. The first is the notion of youth resiliency–the hypothesis that young people, for a variety of reasons, significantly changed their behavior and moved away from involvement in crime, gun violence, and drug use. The second is the notion of community resiliency–the hypothesis that communities, as well as young people, rallied their internal resources to save their neighborhoods from the onslaught of violence. These two possible contributors to the decline in crime, if demonstrated through research, might hold important lessons for those seeking to capitalize on the good news of crime's decline to achieve even greater levels of safety. We examine each of them in turn.

Youth Resiliency

The data are clear: Young people led the way in the great crime reductions of the 1990s. Between 1994 and 2000, arrests of juveniles (under age 18) for murder dropped by 68 percent. Robbery arrests for juveniles were down 51 percent. Arrests for burglary fell by 33 percent (Butts & Travis, 2002). Clearly, the coming "tidal wave of youth violence" did not materialize as had been predicted.

Even more interesting is the fact that the declines in youth violence that began in 1994 were steeper than the rise in youth violence had been during the previous decade. Between 1980 and 1994, juveniles accounted for 19 percent of the increase in arrests for violent crimes, but between 1994 and 2000 they accounted for 33 percent of the decline. Young adults (between 18 and 24 years old) accounted for 13 percent of the rise in violent crime arrests, but accounted for 25 percent of the decline. Taken together, we see this startling fact: Young people (those under 24) were responsible for 32 percent of the increase in violent crime arrests between 1980 and 1994, but accounted for 58 percent of the subsequent drop in arrests between 1994 and 2000. Not only had America not been overrun by superpredators, young people had actually set the pace for the sharpest and longest reductions in violence that the country had ever seen (Butts & Travis, 2002).

We also have some evidence supporting the assertion that juvenile drug use, particularly among the population of young people involved in the criminal justice system, also declined. In 1988, at the height of crack epidemic, 70 percent of defendants between the ages of 18 and 20 who had been arrested and held in police custody in Manhattan tested positive for cocaine, according to reports from the Arrestee Drug Abuse Monitoring (ADAM) program. By 1996, the level of positive tests for cocaine had dropped to 22 percent, a stunning reversal in a very short time. All around the country, other ADAM sites reported similar marked shifts in cocaine use among young people, signaling the end of the crack epidemic (Golub & Johnson, 1997). Again, young people had led the way as hard-pressed communities fought to resist the ravages of the crack trade.

What is less certain is the combination of forces that produced these pronounced shifts in the behavior of young people. Ric Curtis, an anthropologist who lives in and writes about Williamsburg, Brooklyn, has documented a distinct pattern as young people reject the risky behavior of their slightly older siblings (Curtis, 1998). The popular media has dubbed this phenomenon "the younger brother syndrome." In Curtis' observations, a young person growing up in difficult circumstances who sees his older brother involved in drug use and crime, getting arrested, showing the damaging physical effects of crack use, or otherwise seriously off track or anti-social and self-destructive, in essence says to himself, "I won't follow that path." Within the short space of a few years, a tipping point was reached. Young people had demonstrated their resiliency.

Community Resiliency

The theory of community resiliency was perhaps best articulated by Roger Conner, a community activist who organized his northwest Washington, DC, neighborhood to take back the streets from drug dealers. Night after night, he and his neighbors patrolled the streets wearing orange hats, confronted drug dealers and buyers, and worked with the police to report the location of drug stashes and suspicious behavior. They were mobilized into action when patrons of a local drug-dealing bar began firing handguns into the air at closing time on weekends. He once described the spontaneous creation of the Orange Hats, as they were known, as something akin to the "release of the antibodies." Just as antibodies react to the introduction of a disease into the body, so too healthy forces in devastated communities all around the country mustered their collective strength to fight back against the unhealthy forces that were threatening their security (Conner, 1991).

George Kelling, a professor of criminal justice at Rutgers University and co-author of the influential article that coined the phrase "broken windows" (Kelling & Wilson, 1982), described a similar phenomenon in a lecture sponsored by the National Institute of Justice. Asked whether the police department should get all the credit for the stunning decline in crime in New York City, Kelling, a knowledgeable observer of crime and neighborhood patterns in that city, gave credit to the resiliency of communities. Kelling stated that the first signs of a return to safety in the early 1990s in New York City were the spontaneous emergence of tenant organizations, business improvement districts, block watchers, and safety coalitions, all coalescing around the need to reduce crime and restore orderliness to their neighborhoods. Kelling observed that these organizations were then met by a police department with a new focus on community policing–one that was more flexible, receptive and effective in responding to crime conditions (Kelling, 1997). The situation in New York City, where homicides reached an unprecedented level exceeding 2,000 deaths in 1990, was rescued, in part, by the strength of community groups who rallied to save their neighborhoods. The antibodies had fought back.

This general phenomenon has been captured by the image of the "tipping point," a moment in time where the body politic begins to reverse a trend toward unhealthy behaviors and reasserts healthy behaviors (Gladwell, 2000). The anecdote of Roger Conner and the observations of George Kelling also find support in the work of two economists at the University of California, George Akerlof and Janet Yellen. They have developed a complex economic model showing that community resiliency is a key ingredient in fighting crime (Akerlof & Yellen, 1994). What is less clear is how the mechanics of community resiliency actually function. What are the key ingredients of "community" that provide this catalytic force?

We find strong support in the research literature for the general proposition that strong communities are safe communities. For the past ten years, a team of researchers, led by Felton Earls of the Harvard School of Public Health and Robert Sampson of the University of Chicago, has been conducting an ambitious study called the "Project on Human Development in Chicago Neighborhoods." This study is a long-term inquiry into the relationship between crime, delinquency, family functioning, individual development, and the relationships between community members. At the community level, the project has surveyed more than 8,700 adult residents in 343 neighborhoods in Chicago, asking residents about community and family life.

In August 1997, this research team published a groundbreaking article in *Science* magazine (Sampson, Raudenbusch, & Earls, 1997). They reported that the most powerful predictor of violent crime rates is what they termed "collective efficacy"–a term they used to mean a sense of trust, common values and cohesion in a neighborhood. They found the lowest rates of violence in those neighborhoods with a strong sense of community and values, where adults were more likely to intervene in the lives of young people in the community–to step in when children are missing from school, or scrawling graffiti on building walls.

This finding of collective efficacy is important standing alone, but is doubly important when placed in context. Collective efficacy is a stronger predictor of low rates of violence than the racial or ethnic composition of the neighborhood, poverty levels, or the level of residential instability. The ability of a community to work well, particularly in caring for the well-being of its young people, is a powerful and independent force for safety.

The Chicago team has continued to look at the data they collected, in order to unpack this concept of collective efficacy. At the 2001 conference of the American Society of Criminology, they presented some of the more recent findings that provide even more specific context and richness to the relationships between social networks and safety. They asked whether neighborhood factors could explain the levels of individual violence among 12- and 15-year-old males, and found that high levels of "reciprocated exchange" in the neighborhood where the young person lived significantly reduced the likelihood that a young person would engage in violence (Sampson et al., 2001).

By "reciprocated exchange," they refer to simple things like neighbors doing favors for each other, watching each other's children, helping with shopping, lending household tools, and other small acts of kindness. They asked whether residents had parties or get-togethers where other people in the neighborhood were invited. They asked whether neighbors watched over each other's property when their neighbors were not home. When the answers to these questions were positive, there was a high level of "reciprocated exchange," and the young men in that neighborhood were less likely to be engaged in violence. Again, as with the finding regarding collective efficacy, this correlation exists independent of other social factors such as the age, race or socioeconomic status of the youth of the neighborhood.

This research underscores the importance of activities that fall under the broad umbrella of "community building." These findings indicate that social networks can change neighborhoods. If these theories are right, then the message for social policy is clear: Building strong communities "from the ground up"–communities where the "collective" is "efficacious," where neighbors look out for neighbors and everyone cares for the community's young people–will contribute to the reduction in violence and fear, and will create a sense of safety. Coupled with the research evidence demonstrating that young people led the decline in violence in the 1990s, we have an intriguing proposition, namely that organizing a community to help young people grow up safely has a double benefit. These activities strengthen a community's sense of self by reaffirming the importance of young people and underscoring a critical common value. They also help young people to learn to be responsible adults and avoid the risks posed by life in a society with still too many guns, too much temptation to engage in drug use and other risky behaviors, and too much violence.

LESSONS FROM COMMUNITY POLICING INNOVATIONS

If we accept the suggestion from this research that strong communities are safe communities, then we should ask whether partnerships between communities and the police, the governmental agency assigned principal responsibility for responding to crime, can also reduce crime? We quickly discover that there is a significant related issue, namely the level of alienation between the police and the communities they serve, particularly communities of color.

The issue of the legitimacy of the police in the eyes of the public is critical to the broader social challenge of creating a just society (Sherman, 2002). In a just society, the public should believe that the response to crime by the agencies of justice, including the police, is proportional, fair, effective, and tailored to the needs of the community. To ask an alienated community to work with the police to reduce crime is unlikely to be successful, so a discussion of the role of communities in reducing crime must include a discussion of the issue of public trust and confidence in the agencies of justice.

Public Trust and Confidence in the Police

To unpack these related issues, we turn again to lessons learned from the remarkable period of declining crime rates in America. Interestingly, public confidence in the overall performance of the police has not changed much over the past decade, even though crime rates have dropped sharply. In 1993, about 52 percent of the American public reported they had either "a great deal" or "quite a lot" of confidence in the police. That rose to 60 percent in 1996, and then dropped back to 54 percent in 2000. By contrast, the percent of Americans saying they had "a great deal" or "quite a lot" of confidence in "the ability of police to protect them from violent crime" rose from 48 percent in 1989 to 62 percent in 2000.

Apparently, the public is making an important distinction between the crime-fighting abilities of the police and overall police performance. When we try to understand the complexity of police-community relations, there is a striking racial divide. African-Americans have about half the level of confidence in the police as whites. African-Americans are twice as likely as whites to believe there is racial brutality in their neighborhoods. Forty-two percent of African-Americans say they have even been stopped by the police because of their race, compared to six percent of whites.

When we dig deeper, we discover some new twists on the traditional view of the historically troubled relationships between the police and communities of color. The researchers studying the neighborhoods in Chicago have shown that high levels of dissatisfaction with police are determined more by neighborhood poverty and instability than by the racial makeup of the communities. Whites living in disadvantaged, high crime areas are just as hostile toward the police as nonwhites (Sampson et al., 1997).

Researchers at the Vera Institute of Justice in New York City have documented another important determinant of public confidence in the police–powerlessness. The researchers examined a multi-ethnic, predominantly middle-class neighborhood in Queens that had both long-standing ethnic communities as well as new immigrant groups. They found that one's confidence in the police depends on whether one's racial or ethnic community is empowered, meaning that they are represented in local politics and that politicians respond to their needs (Davis, 2000).

According to the Vera study, in communities with a low sense of empowerment, people are less likely to believe the police are effective and more likely to believe the police engage in misconduct. People in these communities are also less likely to report crimes, to talk with the police about neighborhood problems, or talk with the police at all. Contrary to stereotypical views of police-community relations, the two groups with the most positive view of the police were the Italian and African-American communities. In this community, these two groups had a strong sense of political empowerment (Davis, 2000).

Respect is another important dimension of the strength of police-community relations. Tom Tyler, a psychologist at New York University, has studied the enforcement of the law in a variety of settings. His basic research question is, "Why do people obey the law?" According to Tyler, people who feel that they are treated fairly by the police–meaning that the police officer explains the reasons for his actions, does so in a respectful manner, and gives the citizen the opportunity to be heard–have greater confidence in the police. This finding does not depend on the severity of the enforcement action. Just as important, Tyler found that people treated respectfully by the police are also more likely to obey the law in the future (Tyler, 1990). This powerful finding cuts across racial groups, giving strong support to those who argue that respectful policing is good policing. Respectful police officers not only build confidence in the law, they also reduce misconduct in the future.

If police agencies across the country embraced the lessons from this line of research, and could improve trust in the police, that would be a socially valuable result. Other strategies are suggested by this research. Finding ways to enhance the political involvement of marginalized communities is an important goal, with unexpected benefits in terms of public confidence in the police. Working to overcome the racial divide remains a critical challenge. But, pursuit of an agenda of "respectful policing" would seem to have large scale pay off in terms of the relationship between the police and the public.

Yet, there are broader lessons from the policing literature, lessons that shed light on the relationships between communities and other agencies of the criminal justice system. To move our discussion forward, we turn next to a review of a recent, promising reform effort, and the movement to shift the police function toward "community policing." Having seen that community and youth resiliency are untapped assets in society's efforts to produce safety, we ask whether the agencies of justice can be called upon to work more effectively with communities.

Community Role in Community Policing

One of the most trumpeted innovations in American policing has been the concept of "community policing." This policing philosophy is based on two key ideas. First, under the community policing ideal, the police are expected to engage in problem solving, not just crime fighting. In short, the police should examine the contexts and attributes of crime situations, design strategies to address those factors to reduce the incidence of crime, and constantly update and revise their strategies to ensure effectiveness. Second, the police are expected to work in close partnerships with the community. These partnerships are more than a community relations effort. The community is envisioned as a critical player in identifying the crime problems to be addressed, devising strategies to be deployed, and monitoring, with the police, the effectiveness of these strategies.

Thus formulated, the community policing philosophy is a far cry from the notion of the "thin blue line," the concept of the police as the last line of defense between the public and the criminal element. Rather, crime is seen as a problem deeply embedded in communities, a problem that can better be addressed by active, mutual engagement of the police and the affected community.

We have seen in the previous discussion that respectful policing can improve public confidence in the law and can reduce misconduct. But what evidence is there that the engagement of the community in the community policing innovation can reduce crime?

The community policing reform is aptly described as a "movement." The intellectual roots of community policing can be traced to a few critical events in the history of policing in America. In 1974, the Police Foundation released a research report, "The Kansas City Preventive Patrol Experiment," that challenged the prevailing wisdom of police operations. The report found that random, motorized patrol, the prevailing method for assigning police officers, did not reduce crime or fear (Kelling, Pate, Dieckman, & Brown, 1975). Another Police Foundation study, "The Newark Foot Patrol Experiment," found that foot patrol reduced fear of crime and increased community confidence with police (Police Foundation, 1981). The publication of Herman Goldstein's pivotal article, "Improving Policing: A Problem Oriented Approach," in 1979, challenged the profession to adopt "crime problems" rather than "criminal incidents" as the unit of work for police agencies (Goldstein, 1979). In 1985, the Kennedy School of Government launched a multi-year executive session at Harvard, bringing together police chiefs, researchers, community leaders and others to explore the implications of this intellectual ferment for the police function in America. In 1984, the New York City Police Department embarked on the Community Patrol Officer Program, a joint enterprise between the Department and the Vera Institute of Justice, designed to test the twin concepts of problem solving policing and community engagement in a real world environment. Soon, the police profession was abuzz with new ideas, energy, and challenges to the status quo. "Community policing" had been born.

Several large police departments embarked on community policing initiatives. In the presidential contest of 1992, candidate Bill Clinton touted community policing and promised, if elected, to provide federal funding for communities that moved toward this new concept. Following the election, Congress appropriated $9 billion dollars, President Clinton promised that 100,000 police officers would be hired, and that community policing would take hold in American communities. Between 1997 and 1999, the percentage of local police departments with community policing programs increased from one-third to nearly two-thirds (Hickman & Reaves, 2001). By 1999, all large cities in the United States had embraced community policing.

But from city to city, the concept was implemented differently (Roth & Ryan, 2000). Most departments increased their outreach to community groups. Many increased foot patrol or bicycle patrol, in the belief that this policing tactic would increase interaction between the police and community residents, and soften some of the image of the police as an outside force. A smaller percentage of these departments formed active problem-solving partnerships with the community, the "gold standard" of the community policing ideal.

Chicago is home to one of the nation's most ambitious community policing initiatives. Called the Chicago Alternative Policing Strategy, or CAPS, this effort has also produced the most extensive research on the benefits, costs and challenges of implementing community policing. The evaluation, conducted by a team led by Wes Skogan of Northwestern University, resulted in a number of findings central to this discussion of the community's role in producing safety and justice, and the role of the police in working with an engaged community (Skogan & Hartnett, 1997).

First, the CAPS evaluation showed that community policing could reduce crime. This was not a strong finding. In some of the experimental districts where community policing was first introduced in Chicago, crime rates went down faster than would be expected. In others, crime rates did not go down any faster (Skogan, Hartnett, DuBois, Comey, Twedt-Ball, & Gudell 2000). Given the broad scale nature of the community policing innovation, which is typically introduced on a citywide basis, not in a controlled fashion, as was the case in Chicago, we may never be able to get a better answer to the question, "Does community policing reduce crime?"

In many ways, the research findings on the power of community engagement are more illuminating than the inconclusive results on the question whether CAPS reduced crime. For example, the CAPS evaluation suggests that the police could improve public confidence by engaging the community. One of the indicators measured by the evaluation team was police "visibility"–not just police riding in patrol cars, but the presence of the police at community meetings, on foot patrol and talking with community residents. The CAPS evaluation showed that the percentage of people who thought the police were doing a good job rose as a function of how many times they saw police engaged in community-oriented activities. This connection between confidence and visibility held true across all racial groups (Skogan & Hartnett, 1997).

The CAPS evaluation also addressed one of the frequent criticisms of community policing. Opponents of community policing often suggest that this policing philosophy disfavors poor neighborhoods–that the community engagement model may "work" in middle class or stable neighborhoods, but is less likely to "work" in poor neighborhoods with high crime rates. The suggestion is that there is "no community" in impoverished neighborhoods–or people there haven't the time or positive feelings towards the police necessary to be engaged in problem-solving activities. Skogan and his colleagues found just the opposite was true. Attendance at community beat meetings, where police and residents talk about crime problems facing the community, was actually highest in some of the city's poorest and most crime-ridden neighborhoods. In fact, attendance was highest in predominantly African-American neighborhoods.

The bottom line of the CAPS evaluation is very encouraging for those who see community policing as an approach that will improve the standing of the police in the eyes of the public. Over a five-year period, public ratings of the police in Chicago increased by 12 to 20 percentage points along three measures–responsiveness, effectiveness and demeanor. These increases cut across racial groups and social class. The implication is clear–a commitment to a policing philosophy that seeks active engagement of the community will be met by a community eager for that engagement, and the level of trust and confidence between the police and the community will be significantly enhanced.

THE IMPACT OF AMERICAN INCARCERATION POLICIES

Any discussion of the intersection between community life and the workings of our system of laws must recognize that we have paid a heavy price for the popular demand for stricter punishment of those who violate the laws. Over the past generation, we have increased fourfold the per capita rate of imprisonment in this country. Some simple, yet striking statistics document this development:

- In 1973, approximately 110 of every 100,000 Americans were in prison serving a sentence of a year or more. By 1999, that rate reached 476 per 100,000, an increase greater than fourfold.
- These rates of incarceration vary enormously by race. In 1999, one in every 29 African-American males was sentenced to at least a year in prison, compared to one in 75 Hispanic males and one in every 240 Caucasian males.
- The increases in incarceration affect families, as well as children. In the 1990s, the number of minor children with a parent in prison increased from one million to 1.5 million. At the turn of the cen-

tury, two percent of all minor children in the United States had a parent in prison. For African-American children, seven percent had a parent in prison.

- Expenditures on state correction agencies have increased significantly, from $9 billion in 1982 to $44 billion in 1997 (Travis, Solomon, & Waul, 2001).

One consequence of the increase in imprisonment is an increase in the number of people leaving prison. At the turn of the century, well over 600,000 individuals leave our state and federal prisons each year, over 1,600 a day. This is a fourfold increase over the 150,000 who made similar journeys a quarter century ago (see Figure 3).

In important ways, the phenomenon of prisoner reentry is quite different today. More prisoners are returning home having spent longer time in prison, with less preparation for the challenges of reintegration, and with less support and supervision once they are back on the outside (Lynch & Sabol, 2001). One terrible price we have paid for a generation of prison construction and sentencing reform is that we have forgotten what might be called the "iron law" of imprisonment–with the rare exceptions of those who are executed or die from natural causes while in prison, everyone we send to prison returns home.

There is another consequence we have chosen to ignore. These significant increases in the use of imprisonment as a response to crime have penetrated deeply into the fabric of community life in America. Several researchers have now begun to document the consequences of incarceration, as seen through a community lens. For example, if one examines data on the residences of the individuals sent to jail or prison, one can begin to understand the impact of imprisonment at the block level. Predictably, some blocks in urban America "send" disproportionately high numbers of individuals (mostly men) to be housed in America's far-flung network of prisons and jails. Yet, the sheer magnitude of these local effects is staggering. According to an analysis conducted in Brooklyn, New York, there are city blocks where one out of eight parenting-age men is admitted to jail or prison each year.[2] Another analysis conducted in Cleveland, Ohio, found that in that city's neighborhoods where the incarceration effects are felt most acutely, between 8 and 15 percent of the young African-American men are incarcerated on a given day (Lynch & Sabol, 2001).

The consequences of these policies for the communities hardest hit are almost beyond comprehension. What does it mean to grow up in a neighborhood where, if you are a young boy, there is such a high likeli-

FIGURE 3. Sentenced Prisoners Admitted and Released from Federal and State Prison, 1977-98

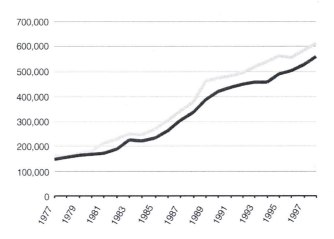

Source: The Urban Institute, 2001. Based on BJS National Prisoner Statistics.

hood that you and many of your peers will go to jail or prison? What does it mean, if you are a girl, to realize that the young men of your neighborhood are often in and out of prison? What does it mean for so many children to be raised by grandparents? What does it mean for the economies of these already impoverished communities to have so many men (and an increasing number of women) sent to prison during the years when they should be learning a trade, establishing a work identity, providing for self and family? These costs–profound social costs–have not been captured by the arid accounting of the cost of a prison cell.

Scholars and practitioners have recently embraced a "reentry perspective" to deconstruct the effects of the growth in imprisonment in America (*Crime and Delinquency,* 2001; Travis, 2001). This framework views sentencing and corrections policies from the perspective of the individuals who pass through America's prisons, their families, and their communities. The reentry perspective looks beyond traditional debates over the wisdom of criminal sentences to explore the world of "invisible punishment"–the collateral consequences of imprisonment (Mauer & Chesney-Lind, 2002).

This perspective compels us to face the realities of reintegrating millions of ex-offenders into modern American society. For the purposes of our discussion about the relationship between our criminal justice policies and communities, the critical question is whether the increase in imprisonment has adversely affected the power of social networks to change neighborhoods. Recalling the earlier description of the finding of "collective efficacy" in the Chicago research project, we could ask whether a fourfold increase in imprisonment–and even greater increases in poor neighborhoods–has weakened the ability of the collective to be efficacious. And, if the answer is yes, what does this portend for the hopeful developments in community engagement that we discussed in connection with the decline in crime rates and the community policing experiment?

The easy answer to the question is yes–sharp increases in the rate of imprisonment have weakened community capacity. But we should not rush to embrace the easy answer. Responding to crime often involves making arrests for violation of the law, and those arrests often lead to prison sentences. In many of the community meetings that form the foundation for community policing, neighborhood residents demand that arrests be made, knowing that imprisonment will follow, and express gratitude when the police do precisely that.

But recent research suggests that this reliance on imprisonment as a response to crime has taken its toll. A team of researchers at the City University of New York, Dina Rose and Todd Clear, have examined the relationship between crime rates and incarceration rates at the community level. They found, as the preceding vignette predicted, that crime decreased as incarceration rates increased. But, very importantly, they found that these effects were short-lived. After a certain percentage of the population had been put into prison, the crime rates went up. A kind of "tipping point" had been reached, they hypothesized, at which the costs outweighed the benefits (Clear, Rose, & Ryder, 2001). At this point, the high rate of incarceration dug too deeply, weakening rather than strengthening the natural ability of a community to fight crime. To borrow Roger Conner's metaphor again, the antibodies could not longer do their jobs, the body had more difficulty fighting back.

The findings of the Rose and Clear research are far from definitive–certainly more research needs to be done to determine whether these early results withstand the rigor of replication. But the hypothesis itself is thought provoking. From one perspective, the suggestion that incarceration has so weakened communities that their natural crime fighting abilities are diminished spells bad news for those committed to community building. Unless our incarceration policies change dramatically–a result not visible on the political horizon–how can we build the capacity of communities to do what communities should do? But the more complicated challenge is to move beyond the simple description of the consequences of incarceration for our communities to ask what relationship should exist between communities and the agencies of justice, particularly the courts and corrections agencies? To borrow from the earlier discussion of the relationship between the police and the community, we should ask whether communities could develop systems of mutual accountability with the courts and corrections agencies? We turn to that question with some reflections on the journey traveled in this chapter.

THOUGHTS ON THE FUTURE OF COMMUNITY ENGAGEMENT ON CRIME AND JUSTICE

Communities can have a powerful role to play in producing an America that is both safer and more just. The community role in producing safety has been well-documented, both in our folklore about the role of community organizations in fighting back against the ravages of the crack epidemic and in our research on "collective efficacy." We have seen promising signs that a police agency that engages the community can strengthen relations between the police and the policed, a relationship critical to the rule of law and to our democracy. We have also seen that respectful policing is itself an effective strategy for enhancing public trust.

The more difficult question is what role communities can play in rolling back the high rates of incarceration. This question is particularly challenging, given the seeming intransigence of the current levels of imprisonment. Yet, I am optimistic that communities can play an important role in reframing this national discussion on the use of prisons. I am fortunate to be leading a team of researchers at the Urban Institute that is developing a national initiative on prisoner reentry. We are working in a number of communities around the country to document the reentry process, and to develop a deeper understanding of the impact of incarceration on prisoners, their families, and their communities. We are finding that there is a refreshing willingness to embrace new ways of thinking about these issues–that some of the most innovative thinking is coming from those experiments that have actively engaged the communities most affected by our high rates of incarceration.

In cities around the country, community groups are becoming engaged in discussions on prisoner reentry. They are asking their justice system who is coming home from prison, when are they returning, and how have they been prepared for reintegration into community life? Leaders from the faith community are playing a particularly important role, asking profound questions about the need for repentance, reconciliation and forgiveness. Business leaders are actively working inside the prison walls, interviewing prisoners as potential future employees. Housing groups are developing new forms of transitional housing for returning prisoners who have no home that can accept them back. In its "Going Home" programs, the federal government has allocated over $100 million in 2002 to fund reentry initiatives in virtually every state around the nation.

In my optimistic moments I believe we are witnessing another "tipping point"–another release of the antibodies–that communities, at some deep level, are saying that the current situation is fundamentally unhealthy. At some level, these community leaders–and their counterparts in government, in the nonprofit sector, and in the philanthropic community–are saying that justice and fairness demand a more proportionate response to the incidence of crime.

Where might this new community interest in the challenges of prisoner reentry be headed? I offer some intriguing possibilities, all within reach. Drawing on the lessons from the community policing experience, can we imagine a set of meetings where community organizations meet around a problem-solving table with police, prosecutors, corrections officials, perhaps even judges and defense lawyers, to set clear expectations for how the justice system should respond to crime? Could the participants in this community conversation agree that the response to crime should be both creative and effective, achieving tangible results in crime reduction while meeting the needs of victims, offenders, and community alike? Could this community group agree that, if there is a decision to deprive someone of his liberty, one of the most profound decisions our government can make, then it should not be made without careful thought, including consideration of the alternatives? Could the community agree that if someone is sent to prison, everyone should start planning for his eventual return in a way that reduces the chance he will cause further harm and increases the chance he will live as a productive citizen? This experiment in problem solving, called by some the "community justice" experiment, can be seen in pockets of innovation around the country (Clear & Karp, 1999).

To make these partnerships work, they would have to be emboldened to ask difficult questions, ones that inherently challenge the orthodoxy of our times–questions about our reliance on punishment as the answer to crime, arrests as the response to a problem, imprisonment as a way to move troublesome and troubled people out of a community. But, perhaps this is the time in our country when those questions can be openly discussed. Now, with the prison building boom apparently over and crime rates at the lowest level in a generation, perhaps we can have a more honest debate. If the debate takes place in the glare of public opinion, or in an election campaign, we are unlikely to make any headway. But, if the ideas and innovations come from problem-solving tables in communities around the country, from the ground up, then we have a chance that the next decade will end with less crime and fewer people in prison.

NOTES

1. Interestingly, rates of property crime in America have been declining steadily since the 1970s. By the turn of the century they had dropped by half, reaching levels lower than those found in most European countries. This good news has not received much attention in the scholarly literature nor in the public debate over crime in America. See Travis and Waul (2002).
2. Analysis by E. Cadora and C. Swartz for The Community Justice Project at the Center for Alternative Sentencing and Employment Services (CASES), 1999. For more information, see *http://communityjusticeproject.org/*.

REFERENCES

Akerlof, G., & Yellen, J. (1994). Gang behavior, law enforcement, and community values. New York: The Brookings Institute.

Blumstein, A. (1995). Violence by young people: Why the deadly nexus? *National Institute of Justice Journal*, 229, 2-9.

Blumstein, A., & Wallman, J. (2000). The recent rise and fall of American violence. In A. Blumstein & J. Wallman (Eds.), *The crime drop in America* (pp. 1-12). New York: Cambridge University Press.

Butts, J., & Travis, J. (2002). *The rise and fall of American youth violence: 1980-2000*. Washington, DC: The Urban Institute.

Clear, T., & Karp, D. (1999). *The community justice ideal: Preventing crime and achieving justice*. Boulder: Westview Press.

Clear, T., Rose, D., & Ryder, J. (2001). Incarceration and the community: The problem of removing and returning offenders. *Crime & Delinquency*, 47(3), 224-351.

Conner, R. (1991). *The winnable war: A community guide to eradicating street drug markets*. Washington, DC: American Alliance for Rights & Responsibilities.

Crime and Delinquency (2001). 47(3): 291-313.

Curtis, R. (1998). The improbable transformation of inner-city neighborhoods: Crime, violence, drugs, and youth in the 1990s. *The Journal of Criminal Law and Criminology*, 88(4), 1223-1276.

Davis, R. (2000). *The use of citizen surveys as a tool for police reform*. New York: The Vera Institute of Justice.

Eck, J., & McGuire, E. (2000). Have changes in policing reduced violent crime? An assessment of the evidence. In A. Blumstein & J. Wallman (Eds.), *The crime drop in America* (pp. 207-265). New York: Cambridge University Press.

Gladwell, M. (2000). *The tipping point: How little things can make a big difference*. New York: Little, Brown, & Company.

Goldstein, H. (1979). Improving policing: A problem oriented approach. *Crime and Delinquency*, 25(2), 236-258.

Golub, A., & Johnson, B. (1997). *Crack's decline: Some surprises among U.S. cities* (Contract No. 95-IJ-CX-0028). Washington, DC: National Institute of Justice.

Hickman, M., & Reaves, B. (2001). Community policing in local police departments, 1997 & 1999. Washington, DC: Bureau of Justice Statistics.

Kelling, G. (1997, November). Crime control, the police, and the cultural wars: Broken windows and cultural pluralism. Paper presented at Perspectives on Crime and Justice Lecture Series. Washington, DC: National Institute of Justice.

Kelling, G., Pate, T., Dieckman, D., & Brown, C. (1975). *Kansas city preventive patrol experiment: A technical report*. Washington, DC: The Police Foundation.

Kelling, G., & Wilson, J. (1982). Broken windows. *The Atlantic Monthly*, 249(3), 29-38.

Lynch, J., & Sabol, W. (2001). *Prisoner reentry in perspective*. Washington, DC: The Urban Institute.

Mauer, M., & Chesney-Lind, M. (Eds.). (2002). *Invisible punishment: The collateral consequences of mass imprisonment*. New York: The New Press.

National Crime Victimization Survey (1973). Washington, DC: Office of Justice Programs.

The Newark foot patrol experiment (1981). Washington, DC: The Police Foundation.

Roth, J., & Ryan, J. (2000). *The COPS program after 4 years–national evaluation* (Contract No. 95-IJ-CX-0073). Washington, DC: The National Institute of Justice.

Sampson, R., Raudenbush, S., & Earls, F. (1997). Neighborhoods and violent crime: A multilevel study of collective efficacy. *Science*, 277, 918-924.

Sampson, R. et al. (2001, November). Project on human development in Chicago neighborhoods: Findings from cohort design. Panel Presentation at the American Society of Criminologist 2001 Annual Conference. Atlanta: American Society of Criminologists.

Sherman, L. (2002). Trust and confidence in criminal justice. *National Institute of Justice Journal*, 248, 22-31.

Skogan, W., & Hartnett, S. (1997). *Community policing, Chicago style*. Oxford: Oxford University Press.

Skogan, W., Hartnett, S., DuBois, J., Comey, J., Twedt-Ball, K., & Gudell, J. (2000). *Public involvement: Community policing in Chicago* (Contract No. 94-IJ-CX-0046 and 95-IJ-CX-0056). Washington, DC: The National Institute of Justice.

Travis, J. (2001). But they all come back: Rethinking prisoner reentry. *Corrections Management Quarterly*, 5(3): 23-33.

Travis, J., Solomon, A. L., & Waul, M. (2001). *From prison to home: The dimensions and consequences of prisoner reentry*. Washington, DC: The Urban Institute.

Travis, J., & Waul, M. (2002, August). *Reflections on the crime decline: Lessons for the future?* Proceeding from the Urban Institute's Crime Decline Forum. Washington, DC: The Urban Institute.

Tyler, T. (1990). *Why people obey the law*. New Haven: Yale University Press.

"So Tell Me, Why Do Women Need Something Different?"

M. Susan Galbraith

SUMMARY. There has been a dramatic increase in the number of women in the criminal justice system over the past two decades, creating the need for gender-specific responses and programs in jails, prisons, and community corrections. Systems must adapt to appropriately respond to women and their families. Institutions and community-based organizations must help women to deal with their histories of trauma, violence, and substance abuse. One gender-specific, strength-based, community model for support is presented. *[Article copies available for a fee from The Haworth Document Delivery Service: 1-800-HAWORTH. E-mail address: <docdelivery@haworthpress.com> Website: <http://www.HaworthPress. com> © 2004 by The Haworth Press, Inc. All rights reserved.]*

KEYWORDS. Women and criminal justice system, women and community re-entry, women and community corrections

INTRODUCTION

Today, there are more women in prison and re-entering communities after incarceration than at any other time in the history of the United

M. Susan Galbraith, MSW, is founder and Executive Director, Our Place, DC, 1236 Pennsylvania Avenue SE, Washington, DC 20003 (E-mail: squalbraith@ourplacedc.org).

[Haworth co-indexing entry note]: "So Tell Me, Why Do Women Need Something Different?" Galbraith, M. Susan. Co-published simultaneously in *Journal of Religion & Spirituality in Social Work* (The Haworth Social Work Practice Press, an imprint of The Haworth Press, Inc.) Vol. 23, No. 1/2, 2004, pp. 197-212; and: *Criminal Justice: Retribution vs. Restoration* (ed: Eleanor Hannon Judah, and Rev. Michael Bryant) The Haworth Social Work Practice Press, an imprint of The Haworth Press, Inc., 2004, pp. 197-212. Single or multiple copies of this article are available for a fee from The Haworth Document Delivery Service [1-800-HAWORTH. 9:00 a.m. - 5:00 p.m. (EST). E-mail address: docdelivery@haworthpress.com].

Digital Object Identifier: 10.1300/J377v23n01_11

States. This trend has enormous implications for the future of our society and especially for a whole generation of children who are growing up separated from their mothers. While it is essential to review and alter the damage that has been done by policies that criminalize drug addiction, a critique of our current public policy is not the subject of this paper. This paper will address what can be done to improve a woman's chance for a successful transition back into the community. It will outline an intervention strategy that gives women the power and resources to negotiate in the community after their imprisonment. The strategy is gender-specific, restorative, nimble, and dignified.

Women in U.S. prisons today are disproportionately African-American, have grown up in communities with high rates of homelessness and unemployment, and were unemployed at the time of their arrest. Certain themes emerge as women report their histories. They have tragically high rates of sexual abuse and trauma. They experienced sexual abuse by a family member or relative at a young age and over a long period of time. They have high rates of alcoholism, drug addiction and mental illness. They are mothers of young children and hope to be reunited with their children upon release. The women have typically committed a nonviolent drug related offense, and their offense has often been tied to their relationship with a man. Their imprisonment has forever changed their lives, the lives of their families and communities, and radically altered their futures.

While in prison or jail, the women who had previously lived in conditions of poverty, trauma and violence, often live in overcrowded cells and units, have access to minimal and substandard health care, mental health, and substance abuse treatment. Furthermore, they can experience sexual abuse from prison staff. They are very often imprisoned hundreds of miles from their children and family.

Women are rarely prepared to meet the overwhelming challenges they must face when they come home. And yet, they do come home and they do face those challenges. Some women succeed, and many women return to prison.

Four questions will be addressed in this paper: (1) who are women in the United States correctional system today; (2) how are they prepared to come home when they are released; (3) what can be done to improve their chances for a successful re-entry into the community; and (4) what if anything should we do differently for women than what we do for men? One gender-specific, strength-based, community support model will be described as an alternative to the overwhelmingly punitive and sanctions-based models of intervention all too often employed with women who are incarcerated and newly released to the community.

Who Are the Women in U.S. Prisons, Jails and Under Supervision?

The number of women in the criminal justice system in the United States has been growing at rapid and alarming rates, and rates higher than men. The rate of incarceration has risen from a low of six sentenced women inmates per 100,000 in 1925 to 600 per 100,000 in 2000 (Mauer & Chesney-Lind, 2002). Between 1983 and 1994, the number of sentenced women prisoners under State and Federal custody rose by 230 percent compared to 134 percent for men. Women accounted for about 16 percent of the total corrections population in 1998. Women represent about 21 percent of those on probation, 11 percent of those in local jails, just under 6 percent of those in prisons, and 12 percent of those on parole. About 84,000 women were in prison and more than 950,000 women were under correctional supervision (Greenfield & Snell, 1999).

Women are far more likely than men to be nonviolent offenders. Sixty (60%) percent of women in prison are serving time for drug or property offenses, compared to 41 percent of men. Nearly half of women prisoners have never been convicted of a violent crime (Mauer & Chesney-Lind, 2002).

There are many similarities among female and male prisoners. Most are young, disproportionately African-American, have children, were unemployed at the time of arrest, and for those who were employed had annual incomes of less than $15,000. There are also major differences between male and female prisoners that have implications for women's confinement and release. Women are less likely to have committed a violent crime, more likely to be serving their first sentence, more likely to be the primary caregiver of their children, more likely to suffer from mental illness, especially depression, and far more likely to have experienced sexual abuse and trauma at a young age and over a prolonged period of time (Morash, Byrum, & Koons, 1998).

Many have written about women's pathways to crime. These pathways, too, are gender specific in that they are dramatically influenced by a woman's experience of childhood trauma and ongoing violence and battering. For example, there is compelling evidence linking childhood sexual abuse to girls' delinquency and running away from home (Mauer & Chesney-Lind, 2002).

Race plays a significant factor in who is arrested, convicted, and incarcerated. A disproportionate number of women in state prisons and jails are women of color. While African-Americans make up 13 percent of the population and Hispanic people 12 percent, the two racial groups account for well over one-half of those who are incarcerated. Forty-eight (48%) percent are African American, 15 percent are Hispanic, and 33 percent are White non-Hispanic. Racial disparities in sentencing are further apparent when looking at who is on community supervision and who is incarcerated. Nearly two-thirds of women under probation supervision are white, while nearly two-thirds of women in local jails, State and Federal prisons are African-American, Hispanic, and other races. Hispanic women account for 1 in 7 prisoners in State prisons and nearly 1 in 3 in Federal custody (Greenfield & Snell, 1999).

Contrary to public perceptions, the majority of women in the criminal justice system are high school graduates. About 60 percent of women on probation, 56 percent of those in State prisons, and 73 percent of those in Federal prisons have completed high school. Between 30 to 40 percent of women high school graduates also completed some college (Greenfield & Snell, 1999).

Women typically lived in more difficult economic situations than men before they entered prison, with about 4 in 10 women in State prisons employed before their arrest as compared with nearly 6 in 10 men. About 37 percent of women and 28 percent of men earned less than $600 in the month before they were arrested and nearly 30 percent of women were receiving welfare as compared to 8 percent of men (Greenfield & Snell, 1999).

Most women in prison are mothers and were far more likely than men to have been the primary caretaker of their children before their arrest. Fifty-eight (58%) percent of women in State prisons and 73 percent of women in Federal prisons were the primary caretakers of their children before their incarceration as compared to 36 percent and 47 percent of men (Mumola, 2000). Many more women than men had been living alone with their children before their arrest, underscoring the profound and disproportionate impact of a mother's arrest and incarceration on her children, who lose their primary caretaker when their mother goes to prison.

Another major gender difference is in the disproportionate number of health problems among women in the criminal justice system. For example, the incidence of HIV/AIDS among women in the Federal and State prison population is higher than it is among men and among the general population. In 1999, 3.4 percent of State female prisoners were HIV positive, compared to 2.1 percent of males (Maruschak, 2001).

Additionally, most incarcerated women have substance abuse problems, and women are more likely than men to be serving time for drug offenses (Morash, Bynum, & Koons, 1998; Mumola, 1999). Nationally, more than half of women test positive for illicit drugs at the time of their arrests; in some cities this number is more than three-quarters of women arrestees (Greenfeld & Snell, 1999). About one-half of women in State prisons had been using alcohol, drugs or both at the time they committed the offense for which they were incarcerated. Women reported to be under the influence of drugs more than alcohol, and men reported the reverse pattern (Greenfeld & Snell, 1999).

More than one-half of women in US prisons have some type of psychiatric problem (Siegal, 1998). One study of nearly 1,300 female jail detainees awaiting trial at the Cook County Jail found that more than eighty percent of the women suffered from one or more lifetime psychiatric disorder (Teplin, Abram, & McClelland, 1996). Often their mental health problems were related to past trauma, including incest, rape, physical and sexual abuse (Boyd, 1993; Nelson-Zlupko, Kauffman, & Dore, 1995).

The rate of physical and sexual abuse among female inmates remains high. In a 1999 survey completed by the Bureau of Justice Statistics, 57 percent of State female inmates and 40 percent of Federal female inmates reported being physically and/or sexually abused before incarceration. Forty-seven percent of State female and 32 percent of Federal female inmates had been physically abused and 39 percent of State female inmates and 23 percent of Federal female inmates had been sexually abused (Wolf Harlow, 1999). Most of the abuse occurred before the women reached the age of 18. A history of rape is also prevalent among female inmates. More than 1 in 3 State prisoners and 1 in 5 Federal prisoners reported being a victim of rape or attempted rape prior to incarceration (Wolf Harlow, 1999). And, being victimized by sexual abuse does not stop at the prison doors.

Sexual misconduct by male correctional officers who are responsible for guarding women has been well documented (Smith, 1998; Human Rights Watch Women's Rights Project, 1996). While the Federal Bureau of Prisons and most states have a "zero tolerance" policy for sexual harassment of women by prison guards, sexual misconduct is commonplace. Women are promised or given coveted goods in exchange for sexual contact.

Histories of trauma are associated with high rates of post-traumatic stress disorder (PTSD) (Fullilove, Mellman, & Duncan, 1995). The experience of PTSD is considerably different for women than for men. Cottler's (1992) study of PTSD rates and substance abuse indicated that female gender and cocaine or opiate use were the strongest predictors of both exposure to a traumatic stressor and the subsequent development of PTSD. Failure to recognize, understand, and respond appropriately to a survivor's symptoms may result in re-victimization (Carmen, Rieker, & Mills, 1984; Fullilove, Mellman, & Duncan, 1995). Re-victimization of trauma survivors has been identified as a significant problem for women prisoners where standard interventions to maintain control, such as seclusion and restraint, are frequently used and can have the effect of worsening symptoms (Carmen, Rieker, & Mills, 1984; Galbraith, 1998).

Why Are So Many Women in Prisons and Jails?

Many have written about the explosion of the prison and jail population in the United States. Three reasons cited for the increased incarceration rates are: (1) the passage of legislation requiring mandatory minimum sentences for drug-related offenses; (2) three strikes legislation in many states that impose a fifteen years to life sentence for individuals convicted of their third felony offense; and (3) truth in sentencing laws that require that a person serve at least 85% of their sentence before becoming eligible for parole (Browne & Lichter, 2001; Mauer & Chesney-Lind, 2002). Underlying these policies was and continues to be the belief that if criminals are sent away longer, society will be safer and that being "tough" on criminals will deter crime (Community Resources for Justice, 2001). The consequences of these policies and attitudes are grave for women and their children. More women are spending longer periods of time in prison, separated from their children and families, and then re-entering back into communities without an infrastructure of support to help them to start their lives over again.

How Are Women Prepared to Come Home When They Are Released?

Both women and men face similar and also daunting challenges as they re-enter society after imprisonment. They need jobs, education, housing, health care, and substance abuse treatment (Community Resources for Justice, 2001; Travis, Solomon, & Waul, 2001). They have been living in a world where they have been stripped of all power and are suddenly expected to take charge of their lives. Individuals return, however, to communities where there are few skilled job opportunities, where they face employment and housing discrimination because of their criminal record, where most are now ineligible for public benefits if they have been convicted of a drug-related felony, and where they are forever ineligible to vote, one of the most basic rights of US citizens (Allard, 2002; Legal Action Center, 2001; Allard & Mauer, 2000).

Both women and men coming home from prison are ill prepared for the challenges they face. They have had few visits with their children and families and have been cut off from their communities. Typically, they come home with no money, no identification, no clothing, and little information about where to turn for help. It is stunning how little people have when they come home.

Our Place, DC, a gender-specific, strength-based community organization described in detail later, provides pre- and post-release services to women. Over 1,000 women seen between its founding in October 1999 and July 2002 were asked what specific things they needed help with upon release. The majority identified a need for housing, employment, and clothing as the top three items for which they needed assistance. Transportation tokens and money for identification were next; medical care, addictions treatment, and education followed (Our Place, DC, initial information form data, 2003). Women in the District of Columbia literally walk to Our Place, DC, from the DC Jail. They are frequently released in their prison jumpsuit, with no money and no place to go. Those who actually make it to the door ask for clothing, food, a place to stay, and a chance to start their lives again. For all people coming out of prison, the world they knew before their incarceration has changed. It has changed even if they have just been away for a year or two.

Women re-entering society after incarceration face very specific challenges that are different than for men and in order to be successful, pre- and post-release programs must be designed to address these differences. Women have had experiences that are unique to their gender, including sexual abuse, sexual assault, domestic violence, adolescent pregnancy, and single parenthood. Research points to a link between women's early alcohol and drug use to their experience of physical and sexual abuse (Bloom, 1998). Without a safe place to go upon re-entry, women are especially vulnerable to continued abuse and violence from men and relapsing into a pattern of alcohol and drug use and crime. Again, in the District of Columbia it is common knowledge that pimps prey on women who are released from the DC Jail late at night, providing their only connection back into the community.

While many prisons do have pre-release programs, all too often, the programs operate in a vacuum. Prisons are frequently located far from home. Prison personnel do not have knowledge of the resources and services in the communities where women are returning. They can only give general guidance on issues such as job hunting, resume preparation, money management, and parenting. And even though many women are under supervision when they return to the community, their supervision officers have enormous caseloads and are ill prepared to deal with the level of need women present.

What Can We Do to Improve Re-Entry Success?

Scores of programs are being developed across the country to deal with the thousands of individuals who are now coming home from prison after serving their sentences. Policymakers are scrambling to establish programs that will monitor people as they are released and are worried about the threat to safe communities posed by the numbers of returning "offenders." Federal and State governments are channeling hundreds of millions of dollars into re-entry programs.

What can we expect to emerge from the attention on prisoner re-entry? Hopefully, this new focus on prisoner re-entry provides an opportunity to structure programs that can help women with the major challenges they face when released from prison. If these efforts are to succeed, they must strike the right balance between supervision and services.

The "moment of release" is a time of crisis. What is in front of a woman as she walks out of the door of prison or jail? In many cases, simple things stand in her way of success. As mentioned earlier in the case of Our Place, DC, women are often released at odd hours of the night without money, identification, clothing, housing, jobs, or substance abuse treatment. In a recent report on prisoner re-entry, the Urban Institute's Justice Policy Center describes the "moment of release" as a time "for policy innovations and attention–to develop strategies that build on a short-term bridge during this immediate transition period (Travis, Solomon, & Waul, 2001).

There are simple barriers that prevent successful re-entry, even for women under supervision or in a community corrections program such as a halfway house. For example, in the District of Columbia, women who are transferred to a halfway house from the Federal Bureau of

Prisons (BOP) are required to find a job within 15 days of their transfer. This is a requirement for all women who have been in the BOP, regardless of whether they have served a two year or twenty year sentence. Women receive no support to obtain the required identification to apply for jobs or the transportation and clothing to go to job interviews. And, it costs $30 just to obtain a birth certificate and photo identification. Many employers will not hire a person with a felony record, even if the woman is fully qualified for the job. Women constantly express their fears about finding a job within the short time they are required to do so and report that the pressure can be unbearable. Women also report discriminatory treatment from employers who will not even consider them because of their felony records. If they are lucky, they find a minimum wage job. Then, they are required to turn over 25 percent of their gross income from the minimum wage job for room and board in the halfway house. It is hard to imagine how one would be able to take the steps to independent living under these circumstances. And, it is remarkable how many women actually do transcend the barriers to re-entry and are successful.

A woman who re-enters the community without even the basic necessities faces an overwhelming challenge to survive. Her chances of success could be greatly increased by beginning release planning long before the day she walks out of the prison door.

Developing relationships with women while they are in prison must be a priority since strong and healthy relationships will be central to women's success when they are released back into the community (Finkelstein, 1996; Covington, 1999). Our Place, DC staff starts meeting with women long before their release.

When the program first started, staff immediately established relationships with the wardens of the federal prisons where the majority of District of Columbia women are incarcerated. Staff worked with the wardens and prison staff to design a program for pre-release that would conform with BOP policies and practices and be consistent with Our Place, DC's mission. A quarterly pre-release class has been conducted in two federal and one state prison. Participation in the classes is voluntary and women earn good time credit. A curriculum has been developed and provides information on obtaining identification, preparing resumes, finding employment, housing, medical care, HIV services, substance abuse treatment, mental health and trauma services, and expectations for transfer to community corrections programs, "the halfway house." The same staff has taught the pre-release classes for three years, and this consistency has made it possible for women to develop relationships with specific individuals who are then available for support upon their re-entry.

Recently, Our Place, DC has implemented a two-day HIV peer educator training and certification program for women in prison. The goal of this program is to give women the tools to educate each other about HIV prevention. The certification also gives women a marketable skill for when they are released.

The program also provides monthly transportation for families to visit women in one federal prison located about 6 hours from the District of Columbia, a holiday party for children that is given on behalf of their mothers who are in prison, birthday cards for women, regular written correspondence, and legal services. All family-centered activities are organized through the mother. She is given information, passes it on to families, and the caretakers of her children, and they, in turn, contact the program. This approach restores power to mothers in prison, giving them some authority for their children, and allowing them to be a parent from a distance by making decisions about how their children will participate in the program.

The program's policy is to accept collect calls from women since the costs of phone calls are too often a major barrier to seeking outside help. This policy has proven extremely effective and not nearly as costly as anticipated because it is another way women gain power in an otherwise powerless situation where information is hard to come by, resources are extremely limited, and contact and connection with the outside world is highly restricted.

What Should We Do Differently for Women?

Over the past two decades, a rich literature has developed on gender specific treatment. For example, Bloom has written extensively on the role of gender in corrections. In her 1998 review of the literature, she reviewed the studies of promising programs for women offenders both in prison and in community corrections. While noting the paucity of outcome research on gender specific corrections interventions, she pointed out certain themes common to these programs that prove to be promising. Programs identified as having "promising practices" use an "empowerment" model, working to broaden the range of skills, responses, and coping mechanisms of women. They combine supervision and specialized services to meet the needs of women in structured and "safe" environments.

Gender-specific programs employ a comprehensive and "holistic" model and address women's specific issues, including drug addiction and alcoholism, domestic violence, sexual abuse, pregnancy and parenting, relationships, and gender bias. Others have identified the key elements of a gender specific approach. Gender specific services are not simply "female only" programs that were designed for men. They have very specific elements that define their values and approaches. These programs: (1) are based in the identification of women's strengths, not their limitations or "weaknesses"; (2) avoid a confrontational approach; (3) offer a safe, nurturing and supportive environment; (4) have specific staff and services targeted to serve identified underserved populations of women; (5) address relationship issues, especially love relationships with partners and mothers' relationships with their children; (6) hire staff who can develop authentic, caring, and trusting relationships with women; (7) teach coping strategies, based on women's experiences, with a willingness to explore women's individual appraisals of stressful situations; (8) arrange program hours that can accommodate working women and mothers of school-age children or are coordinated with the local elderly transportation service; (9) promote bonding among women; (10) have a strong female presence on staff; (11) have staff trained to be sensitive to women's issues; and (12) offer women only treatment sessions (Center for Substance Abuse Treatment, 1994; Covington, 1999).

Our Place, DC: A Gender-Specific Re-Entry Model

Our Place, DC offers gender specific services for District of Columbia women who are in prison and newly released. The program model is based on the growing research and practice literature on gender specific services that has been conducted in the substance abuse, trauma, and corrections areas. The organization is a private, nonprofit, community-based organization, and was founded in 1999. The program mission is to women who are or have been incarcerated with the support and resources they need to resettle in the community, reunite with their families, and find decent housing and jobs. The goal of the program is to prevent re-incarceration by providing gender specific, comprehensive support and re-entry programs for women prisoners from the District of Columbia and their families.

Our Place, DC offers an alternative to existing community corrections in that participation is voluntary, and services are delivered based on the identified needs of each woman who requests assistance. No sanctions are imposed on participants and there is no monitoring, surveillance, or oversight function.

Women learn about the program through word of mouth, pre-release classes for which they receive good time credit, and a quarterly newsletter called *Finding Our Place*. Most of the program funding is private from local and national foundations, individuals, businesses, religious organizations, and civic groups.

What makes this program different? Women are given the power to make decisions about their lives and the lives of their children and families. Staff affirms women's strengths and capacities to make decisions for themselves by asking them to make a check-list of their needs and then building a treatment plan based on their check-list. This overall approach is antithetical to the approach of the criminal justice system, in which women are stripped of all power and control and struggle to maintain their identity and sense of self.

From the start, women are empowered when they are given an Initial Information Form in which they identify their service needs. This is the only form women are asked to fill out and filling it out is completely voluntary. Few questions are asked about a woman's past. The focus is on the present, what a woman needs to take the next step in her life, and how Our Place, DC can assist with that step. Women always offer information about their histories, crimes, and families. However, they offer this information after getting to know and trust the staff. The therapeutic relationship is built on respect, trust, and empowerment. Here are some examples of how the program implements this approach.

Building a System of Care

Our Place, DC has worked through a network of community-based programs to develop a high quality system of resources in health care, substance abuse and mental health treatment, family and children's services, transitional housing, and employment. Women and their families have timely access to gender-specific resources through this network that are responsive and where they are treated with dignity. Timely access to high quality services is an important organizational value because all too often, women report negative experiences with care providers in which they have felt looked down upon and discriminated against because of their criminal, addiction, and health issues, especially if the woman is HIV positive. Women report a reluctance to seek care because of the attitudes of providers and the barriers that make it difficult to get what they need. Lack of health insurance, long waiting lists, unresponsive and negative service providers, and bureaucratic red tape have all been identified as barriers to seeking help by women.

For example, service agreements are in place with a community health clinic where women and their families have free and immediate access to health care services. Other service agreements are with outpatient and residential substance abuse treatment programs, family and children's mental health services, legal services, HIV/AIDS treatment, housing and supportive services, and transitional housing programs. Women are only referred to organizations that are known and respected by Our Place, DC staff. In fact, the staff frequently tells women that they "would not send them anywhere they wouldn't go themselves." Long before their release, women are made aware of this continuum of care and the support that they can plan for their re-entry.

Responding Immediately to Basic Needs

Services are provided for women when they are transferred to community corrections' programs (halfway house) or released directly to the community. Women are provided with clothing, money for identification, and transportation tokens. An on-site support group provides a chance for socializing and support from other women who are facing and managing the challenges of re-entry. The support groups provide an opportunity for women to develop relationships with other women in recovery and build a new community of support. One woman described her experience in a focus group on relationships. "Our Place, DC helped me to realize how important relationships are to my recovery. Today my relationships play a major part in me being able to get from one day to the next. I'm able to pick up a phone and call my sponsor, or a friend, or someone at Our Place and say, 'hey my life's messed up right now, I need some help.' It is good to be able to have that connection with someone else. I never had that before."

Ongoing and Long-Term Support

Our Place, DC provides ongoing, long-term support. Some women return home from prison and have no family or community to turn to for support. Our Place, DC becomes "family" for those women who have lost all of their connections. Other women do have family but those families have changed dramatically during their time in prison. Family members have died, marriages and partnerships have dissolved, grandmothers have replaced their daughters as mothers, and children have grown into adults. The program provides support for the whole family through the re-entry transition. This support is especially important when women are reuniting with their children and entering into a family system where their own mother has been mothering their children. There can be enormous tension, resentment, and role confusion during this transition and intensive support and guidance is needed for all mothers, caretakers, and children.

Program Planning and Development

Our Place, DC programs are developed based on the identified needs of incarcerated and formerly incarcerated women and the advice and feedback from women is regularly solicited. An Evaluation Advisory Board of formerly incarcerated women, program staff, and board has designed methods to evaluate the "Educate Your Sisters" program, an HIV/AIDS peer education and certification program. A pre- and post-test, a satisfaction survey, and a three-month follow-up to measure knowledge retention and behavior change are administered. This evaluation model will be extended to other programs in the coming year and is central to the program's commitment to responding to the expressed needs of women through a high-quality, gender-specific system of care.

CONCLUSION

Both women and men who return to society after their imprisonment face enormous challenges as they reintegrate into the community. Often, they must secure housing, employment, health care, legal services, and substance abuse and mental health treatment. Women have additional challenges. They are often in far worse economic situations than men, with no job histories and few job skills. Women more often than men, return home to children who require their immediate care and attention. Many women have histories of abuse and trauma, interwoven with their drug and alcohol addiction, and relationships with abusive partners. They must have the opportunity to deal with their histories of trauma in order to recover from the violence of their past and move forward.

Most importantly, women coming home need an environment where they can be open and honest about their pasts, take responsibility for their actions, and begin to heal. They need an economic base to support their independence and a compassionate guide to help them along the way. The policies that have led to incarcerating women in record numbers have devastated families and communities across the United States. These policies seem a far greater threat to the safety of our communities than the nonviolent drug-related crimes women typically commit. The current focus on "re-entry" provides an opportunity for restorative justice, where women can make amends for their crimes while at the same time, have a real chance to gain the support and resources needed to live a dignified life. When persons walk out of prison after serving their sentence, they have done their time. It is most certainly cruel and unusual punishment to make them and their families pay for the rest of their lives.

REFERENCES

Allard, P. (2002). Life sentences: Denying welfare benefits to women convicted of drug offenses. Washington, DC: The Sentencing Project.

Allard, P., & Mauer, M. (2000). Regaining the vote: An assessment of activity relating to felon disenfranchisement laws. Washington, DC: The Sentencing Project.

Bloom, B. (1998). Beyond recidivism: Perspectives on evaluations of programs for female offenders in community corrections. Arlington, VA: International Community Corrections Association.

Boyd, C. (1993). The antecedents of women's crack cocaine abuse: Family substance abuse, sexual abuse, depression and illicit drug use. *Journal of Substance Abuse Treatment*, 10, 443-438.

Browne, A., & Lichter, E. (2001). Imprisonment in the United States. *Encyclopedia of Women and Gender*, Volume A-K, 611-623. London: Academic Press.

Carmen, E.H., Rieker, P.P., & Mills, T. (1984). Victims of violence and psychiatric illness. *American Journal of Psychiatry*, 141, 378-383.

Center for Substance Abuse Treatment. (1994). Practical approaches in the treatment of women who abuse alcohol and drugs. Rockville, MD: Center for Substance Abuse Treatment.

Community Resources for Justice. (2001). Returning inmates: Closing the public safety gap. Boston, MA.

Cottler, L.B., Compton, W., Mager, D., Spitznagel, E., & Janca, A. (1992). Post traumatic stress disorder among substance abusers in the general population. *American Journal of Psychiatry*, 149 (5), 664-670.

Covington, S. (1999). Helping women recover. San Francisco, CA: Jossey-Bass Publishers.

Finkelstein, N. (1996). Using the relational model as a context for treating pregnant and parenting chemically dependent women. *Journal of Chemical Dependency Treatment*, Vol. 6, No. 12, 23-44.

Fullilove, M.T., Mellman, L., & Duncan, M.W. (1995). Violence against women in the United States: A comprehensive background paper. New York: Commonwealth Fund Commission on Women's Health.

Galbraith, S. (1998). And so I began to listen to their stories: Working with women in the criminal justice system. Delmar, NY: GAINS Center.

Greenfield, L.A., & Snell, T.L. (1999). Women offenders. Bureau of Justice Statistics. Washington, DC: US Department of Justice.

Human Rights Watch Women's Prison Project. (1996). All too familiar, sexual abuse of women in U.S. state prisons. New York, NY: Human Rights Watch.

Legal Action Center. (2001). Getting to work: How TANF can support ex-offender parents in the transition to self-sufficiency. New York, NY: Legal Action Center.

Maruschak, L.M. (2001). HIV in prisons and jails. Bureau of Justice Statistics. Washington, DC: U.S. Department of Justice.

Mauer, M., & Chesney-Lind, M. (2002). Invisible punishment. New York, NY: The New York Press.

Morash, M., Byrum, T., & Koons, B. (1998). Women offenders: Programming needs and promising practices. Research in brief. Washington, DC: National Institute of Justice.

Mumola, C. (2000). Incarcerated parents and their children. Bureau of Justice Statistics. Washington, DC: US Department of Justice.

Mumola, C. (1999). Substance abuse and treatment, state and federal prisoners, 1997. Bureau of Justice Statistics. Washington, DC: US Department of Justice.

Nelson-Zlupko, L., Kauffman, E., & Dore, M.M. (1995). Gender differences in drug addiction and treatment: Implications for social work intervention with substance-abusing women. *Social Work*, 40 (1), 45-54.

Our Place, D.C. Initial information form data, 2003. Unpublished.

Siegal, N. (1998). Women in Prison. *Ms. Magazine* (September/October).

Smith, B.V. (1998). An end to silence: Women prisoners' handbook on identifying and addressing sexual misconduct. Washington, DC: National Women's Law Center.

Teplin, L.A., Abram, K.M., & McClelland, G.M. (1996). Prevalence of psychiatric disorders among incarcerated women. *Archives of General Psychiatry*, 53 (6), 505-512.

Travis, J., Solomon, A.L., & Waul, M. (2001). From prison to home the dimensions and consequences of prisoner reentry. Washington, DC: Urban Institute.

Wolf Harlow, C. (1999). Prior abuse reported by inmates and probationers. Bureau of Justice Statistics Washington, DC: US Department of Justice.

Social Work and Criminal Justice: The Uneasy Alliance

Frederic G. Reamer

SUMMARY. We shall begin with the principal, and complicated, conclusion: Regrettably, the social work profession has largely abandoned the criminal justice field. That is not to say that social workers are not employed in criminal justice settings. Certainly they are. Significant numbers of social workers earn their living as probation and parole officers, caseworkers in public defender offices, counselors in correctional institutions and halfway houses, and so on. As a profession, however, social work no longer has a major presence in the criminal justice field (Gibelman and Schervish, 1993). Relatively few social workers embark on their professional education with the aim of employment in the criminal justice field. Virtually no courses in social work education programs focus explicitly or comprehensively on criminal justice (Knox and Roberts, 2002; McNeece and Roberts, 1997). Workshops offered at professional conferences or continuing education seminars rarely focus on criminal justice issues per se. And, relatively little serious scholarship on criminal justice issues is authored by social workers.

Frederic G. Reamer, PhD, is Professor, School of Social Work, Rhode Island College, Providence, RI 02908 (E-mail: freamer@ric.edu). He has been a member of the State of Rhode Island Parole Board since 1982. Other criminal justice involvement includes serving as a social worker in both state and federal prisons, and in forensic research.

[Haworth co-indexing entry note]: "Social Work and Criminal Justice: The Uneasy Alliance." Reamer, Frederic G. Co-published simultaneously in *Journal of Religion & Spirituality in Social Work* (The Haworth Social Work Practice Press, an imprint of The Haworth Press, Inc.) Vol. 23, No. 1/2, 2004, pp. 213-231; and: *Criminal Justice: Retribution vs. Restoration* (ed: Eleanor Hannon Judah, and Rev. Michael Bryant) The Haworth Social Work Practice Press, an imprint of The Haworth Press, Inc., 2004, pp. 213-231. Single or multiple copies of this article are available for a fee from The Haworth Document Delivery Service [1-800-HAWORTH, 9:00 a.m. - 5:00 p.m. (EST). E-mail address: docdelivery@haworthpress.com].

Interestingly, this has not always been the state of affairs. Earlier in the profession's history, social workers were much more visible and vocal participants in dialogue, debate, research, and practice related to criminal justice. Ideally–in light of social work's unique perspectives on practice and social problems, and the profession's noble value base–the profession will reclaim its preoccupation with criminal justice. As Sarri (2001) concludes with respect to social workers' involvement in the juvenile justice system in particular:

> Thirty years ago, social workers were in leadership positions in juvenile justice in the majority of states. In the 1980s, a gradual decline began in agencies and in social work education for practice in juvenile justice. Some have suggested that the decline was at least partially due to professional resistance to working in coercive settings with involuntary clients. However, given the millions of people now caught up in the criminal justice system who are not receiving the social services they desperately need, it is a priority that social work return to a more central role in criminal justice. (p. 453)

[Article copies available for a fee from The Haworth Document Delivery Service: 1-800-HAWORTH. E-mail address: <docdelivery@haworthpress. com> Website: <http://www.HaworthPress.com> © 2004 by The Haworth Press, Inc. All rights reserved.]

KEYWORDS. Criminal justice, social work education, values, mission

THE EARLY YEARS

When social work was formally inaugurated as a profession in the late 19th century, one of its most noteworthy features was its intense and influential involvement in the criminal justice field, especially with respect to juveniles. The conceptual foundation on which the juvenile justice system was based–that misbehavior typically is a function of the complex interaction among diverse psychological, familial, economical, environmental, and biological factors–was remarkably consistent with the intellectual perspectives that were emerging in the fledgling social work field. It is perhaps no great coincidence that the first juvenile court in the U.S. (Cook County [Chicago] Illinois) and the first formal social work education program (the New York Charity Organization Society training program) were created in the very same year: 1899. That is, in the late 19th century there was a relatively small group of insightful, astute pioneers who recognized that meaningful efforts to assist people in need require a comprehensive, in-depth understanding of human nature and the broader culture. Narrow preoccupation with personality, family, community, economy, policy, and so on, would not suffice; rather, we needed to invent a more integrated approach. Clearly, the marriage between social work and juvenile justice was a natural.

Evidence of social work's values and perspectives dominate the emergence of juvenile justice. Although the social work field was too young in the late 19th century for there to have been explicit references to the profession in prominent juvenile justice publications, the values and concepts that have come to be associated with social work were clearly evident. At the time, consensus was emerging that misbehaving children ought to be "saved" (rehabilitated) and not punished. For example, the Board of Public Charities of the state of Illinois noted in 1879, shortly before the first juvenile court was established, that "the object of reformatory institutions is well stated; it is not punishment for past offenses, but training for future usefulness" (Platt, 1977, p. 106). And in 1899 the year the first juvenile court was created, a delegate to the National Prison Association urged that we should "Point out to the children . . . all that is beautiful in nature and art . . . teach them to love mother and the home, and to hope for heaven . . . Give the little fellows good companionship, decent, comfortable quarters, clean beds and wholesome food. Smile on them, speak to them, and let sunshine into their souls" (Platt, 1977, p. 70). Although this rhetoric seems quaint by today's standards, it clearly reflects the inclination and willingness of the earliest juvenile justice professionals to approach rehabilitation constructively and supportively rather than punitively.

What today's social workers call a "strengths perspective" (Rapp, 1998; Saleebey, 1996, 1997)–which embraces and seeks to enhance human beings' abilities, coping strategies, and resilience rather than focus on disability, dysfunction, disease, and pathology–dominated the earliest writings on the needs of young offenders. For example, soon after the first juvenile court began operation in Cook County, Illinois, its first chief probation officer concluded that:

> Those interested in saving the little ones from the fearful future, which seemed to be yawning for them realized that the fountain-head of the evil, vice and crime as well as of virtue and honor, was to be found in the home surroundings of the child. The wisest efforts to reform abuses were thwarted by homes that were de-

praved. It was realized that the real criminal was not the individual himself, but the entire social body that permitted conditions to exist, which could produce only criminals. (Hurley, 1907, p. 57)

The climate of the time was echoed by the first judge of the court, who commented on his approach to misbehaving youth:

> I first speak to him in a kindly and considerate way, endeavoring to make him feel that there is no purpose on the part of anyone about him to punish, but rather to benefit and help, to make him realize that the State–that is, the good people of the State–are interested in him, and want to do only what will be of help to him now and during his entire life. (Tuthill, 1904, p. 1)

Along the way, the academic literature on crime and delinquency, and their causes, supported the evolving view that offenders' behavior was, to a great extent, a function of structural and environmental forces that needed to be addressed–a point of view quite consistent with social work's. In the early 20th century the works of the Italian positivists–Cesare Lombroso, Enrico Ferri, and Raffaele Garofalo–paved the way for subsequent writings on the physiological, psychological, economical, and environmental determinants of crime and delinquency (Reamer, 2003; Quinney, 1970).

The so-called Chicago school of the 1920s, including Ernest Burgess, Clifford Shaw, and Henry McKay, highlighted ecological factors that were thought to account for most delinquency. Robert Merton's classic analysis in 1938 focused on the complex tension between individuals' goals and the opportunities available to reach them (Sutherland and Cressey, 1966).

As in other social work domains, World War II turned many scholars' and practitioners' attention toward psychiatric and psychodynamic constructs. A number of analyses during the 1940s and 1950s focused on the connection between poor character formation and delinquent behavior (Berman, 1959) and the challenges of adolescent development (Bloch and Niederhoffer, 1958). In 1955, Albert Cohen published his classic Delinquent Boys, in which he explained delinquent behavior as a "reaction formation" against middle-class values, and in 1960 Richard Cloward and Lloyd Ohlin published their very influential book, Delinquency and Opportunity, which examined the influence of social structure on delinquent behavior.

As the justice field developed, so too did the social work profession. Although each field developed its own intellectual traditions, vocabulary, conceptual frameworks, and interventions, there was plenty of opportunity for collaboration and intersection. Before long, social workers were prominent fixtures in reformatories, probation and parole offices, and court services. The professional marriage worked in most respects, at least up through the 1960s and early 1970s.

THE DECLINE

Beginning in the mid-to-late 1960s, public opinion about the challenge of crime and delinquency began to change. These changes introduced some friction between traditional social work values and the goals and mission of the criminal justice field. In May 1965, the Gallup poll reported that for the first time "crime" was listed as the nation's most important problem (Wilson, 1975). This public mood set the stage for a decline in tolerance for programs that emphasized rehabilitation over public safety (Bernard, 1992; Guarino-Ghezzi and Loughran, 1998; Shireman and Reamer, 1986).

In the juvenile justice field, in particular, which historically shared so many of social work's values, there was growing recognition that the lofty goals of rehabilitation were not being realized in traditional correctional programs. Rather, the typical correctional program was far more punitive than most professionals had been willing to acknowledge. The conclusions of the influential President's Commission on Law Enforcement and Administration of Justice (1967), which had been created by President Lyndon Johnson in July 1965 to provide a comprehensive assessment of the nation's crime problem, clearly reveal the growing preference among many for stricter and more formal responses to youthful offenders:

> The limitations, both in theory and in execution, of strictly rehabilitative treatment methods, combined with public anxiety over the seemingly irresistible rise in juvenile criminality, have produced a rupture between the theory and practice of juvenile court dispositions. While statutes, judges, and commentators still talk the language of compassion, help, and treatment, it has become clear that in fact the same purposes that characterize the use of the criminal law for adult offenders–retribution, condemnation, deterrence, incapacitation–are involved in the disposition of juvenile offenders too. These are society's ultimate techniques for protection against threatening conduct; it is inevitable that they should be used

against threats from the young as well as the old when other resources appear unavailing. (President's Commission, 1967, pp. 8-9)

Within a relatively short period of time, the context in which social workers had functioned was shifting. The fit between the values and missions of the social work profession and the justice system was losing its alignment. What were once relatively supportive and hospitable environments for social workers' agendas were becoming less so, and this was occurring at a time when employment options for social workers in other settings were expanding (Gibelman and Schervish, 1993). The sentiments of the President's Commission, which set the national tone, were clearly moving the field in a direction at odds with social work's perspectives, goals, and methods:

The cases that fall within the narrowed jurisdiction of the court and filter through the screen of informal, prejudicial, informal disposition methods would largely involve offenders for whom more vigorous measures seem necessary. Court adjudication and disposition of those offenders should no longer be viewed solely as a diagnosis and prescription for cure, but should be frankly recognized as an authoritative court judgment expressing society's claim to protection. While rehabilitative efforts should be vigorously pursued in deference to the youth of the offenders and in keeping with a general commitment to individualized treatment of all offenders, the incapacitative, deterrent, and condemnatory aspects of the judgment should not be disguised. (1967, p. 2)

Thus began what has turned out to be some cleavage between social work and the criminal justice fields. Although a modest number of social workers continue to work in juvenile and criminal justice settings, very few enter the profession with this goal in mind. Further, social workers employed in juvenile and criminal justice settings sometimes experience the context as one that is hostile toward social work's values and mission; it is not unusual to hear social workers in court and correctional settings complain that their training, education, and goals are neither appreciated nor supported by colleagues whose orientations are more closely aligned with law enforcement and public safety.

The data are compelling. A 1951 survey of social workers (Hollis and Taylor, 1951; Miller, 1995) documented that about 12 percent of practitioners were employed in some aspect of the justice system (juvenile or adult probation, parole, or the courts). Forty years later, Gibelman and Schervish (1993) found that only 1.2 percent of NASW members were employed in jobs related to the justice system. As Miller (1995) concludes, "there are relatively few social workers in corrections who have been trained as such. Instead, the workers tend to have a college degree with occasional graduate courses in counseling" (p. 656).

THE CASE FOR SOCIAL WORK

The unfortunate reality is that the social work and justice fields are no longer integrated in the way they once were. Many juvenile and criminal justice professionals obtain their professional education in allied professions, such as counseling and psychology. The poignant irony, however, is that, at least in principle, social work should be central to the juvenile and criminal justice fields. Social work's longstanding value base, mission, and substantive expertise have much to offer the justice system. The most compelling evidence of this "goodness of fit" resides in the National Association of Social Workers Code of Ethics (1997). The current code–only the third since the inception of NASW–includes a novel and detailed statement of social work's principal mission, values, broad ethical principles, and specific ethical standards. A close reading of the code yields the strongest possible arguments for social work's serious reengagement with the criminal justice field. The Code's Preamble–which was written broadly to pertain to the entire social work profession–asserts that:

> The primary mission of the social work profession is to enhance human well-being and help meet the basic human needs of all people, with particular attention to the needs and empowerment of people who are vulnerable, oppressed, and living in poverty. A historic and defining feature of social work is the profession's focus on individual well-being in a social context and the well-being of society. Fundamental to social work is attention to the environmental forces that create, contribute to, and address problems in living. (p. 1)

If one reads this passage with criminal justice in mind, one can hardly find a better focus for the social work profession. There is no question that offenders, both adults and juveniles, are disproportionately poor, vulnerable, and victims of oppression, such as discrimination based on race, ethnicity, national origin, color, sex, and mental or physical disability. Of course, such traits neither excuse nor justify unacceptable, harmful, and pernicious delinquent and criminal behavior. However, any seasoned professional in the criminal justice field understands that poverty, mental illness, addiction, racism, and other vulnerabilities account for a remarkably large portion of criminal behavior. No other human services profession has formally adopted a mission statement that resembles social work's genuine and enduring commitment to addressing the social problems and circumstances that give rise to these etiological factors.

The Preamble also highlights social work's recognition that individual behavior must be examined and understood by considering the influences of political, economical, geographical, familial, and other structural factors that, to a great extent, shape human behavior. In contrast to the fields of psychology, psychiatry, and counseling, social work has articulated its explicit determination to address individuals' behavior in a social context–a perspective that is essential to any serious attempt to prevent and respond to criminal behavior.

In addition, the Code's Preamble highlights social work's historic commitment to social justice issues, particularly as they pertain to members of minority and otherwise oppressed groups: "Social workers promote social justice and social change with and on behalf of clients . . . Social workers are sensitive to cultural and ethnic diversity and strive to end discrimination, oppression, poverty and other forms of social injustice" (p. 1). Social workers' finely honed advocacy skills are critically important in light of the discrimination, oppression, poverty, and other forms of injustice that lead to crime and delinquency in the first place and that exacerbate its magnitude. Further, social workers' moral obligation to confront social injustice is relevant within the criminal justice field itself, considering documented evidence of discrimination and oppression within the field in the form of, for example, racial and social class bias in recruitment of police, arrest rates, prosecutions, access to legal counsel, prison sentences, referral to community-based diversion programs, and use of capital punishment (Barton, 1995; Bonczar and Beck, 1997; Fagan, Forst, and Vivona, 1987; Iglehart, 1995; Krisberg and Austin, 1993; Mann, 1993; Mauer, 1997; Miller, 1996; National Council of Juvenile and Family Court Judges, 1990; Pope and Feyerherm, 1993; Sarri, 2000; Tonry, 1995).

The NASW Code of Ethics also includes several specific standards concerning social and political action that distinguish the profession from other human services professions. No other human services profession's code of ethics reflects a comparable commitment to social justice. The NASW code's strongly worded mandates highlight the relevance of social work to the administration of a fair and equitable criminal justice system:

> Social workers should engage in social and political action that seeks to ensure that all people have equal access to the resources, employment, services, and opportunities they require to meet their basic human needs and to develop fully. Social workers should be aware of the impact of the political arena on practice and should advocate for changes in policy and legislation to improve social conditions in order to meet basic human needs and promote social justice. (standard 6.04[a])

> Social workers should act to expand choice and opportunity for all people, with special regard for vulnerable, disadvantaged, oppressed, and exploited people and groups. (standard 6.04[b])

> Social workers should act to prevent and eliminate domination of, exploitation of, and discrimination against any person, group, or class on the basis of race, ethnicity, national origin, color, sex, sexual orientation, age, marital status, political belief, religion, or mental or physical disability. (standard 6.04[d])

A RECLAMATION BLUEPRINT

Ideally, social workers should reflect on the current state of affairs in juvenile and criminal justice and reexamine what the profession can contribute in light of its unique aims, purposes, and methods. Social workers should ask two overarching questions in their effort to reclaim their prominence and influence in the juvenile and criminal justice fields. First, in light of significant developments and changes over time in both social work and the justice system, what does social work have to offer considering its practitioners' knowledge, values, and skills? Second, what practical steps might social workers take to enhance their involvement in the justice system?

Social work education is designed to train practitioners to perform a variety of functions in human services settings, including clinical practice, administration, policy practice, supervision, organizing, advocacy, and research and evaluation. Foundation-level education in social work includes content on work with individuals, families, couples, and small groups; human behavior; community and organizational dynamics; social policy; research and evaluation; social, cultural, and ethnic diversity; and values and ethics. Social work education is unique in its broad approach to human services, an approach that seems to be tailor-made for work with adult and juvenile offenders and with the various components of the juvenile and criminal justice systems. In principle, social workers with advanced training are educated to be able to provide clinical and case management assistance to individual offenders and their families; design, administer, and evaluate programs; supervise staff; and advocate and lobby for legislative and other social change.

Beyond their professional knowledge and practical skills, social workers have unique contributions to make to the criminal justice system because of the profession's longstanding and deep-seated values. As noted earlier, this fortuitous, and not entirely coincidental, fit was evident in the late 19th century when both social work and the juvenile court movement got their formal start. Decades later, during the late 1960s, the complementary nature of social work's values and key developments in criminal justice was again clear. Following the release of the report of the President's Commission on Law Enforcement and Administration of Justice–which contained sweeping recommendations and proposals for widespread reforms–the criminal justice field earnestly pursued several major goals that have always garnered strong support among social workers: *due process, diversion, decriminalization,* and *deinstitutionalization.* In criminal justice settings, due process entails protection of clients' legal rights related to, for example, representation by counsel, speedy trials, self-incrimination, and the confrontation of witnesses. The broader subject of clients' rights–for example, related to privacy and confidentiality, protection from harm and exploitation, and participation in the development of intervention plans–has always been central to social work.

Also, social workers have generally favored the diversion of clients from large, potentially toxic, bureaucratic agencies when less formal, community-based programs were available and appropriate (Miller, 1991; Reamer and Shireman, 1981). And, in many instances social workers have preferred that clients who become involved with law enforcement agencies receive services in social service and mental health settings rather than correctional settings, when this is a realistic option (Singer, 1996). Thus, the general tenor of reforms that dominated juvenile and criminal justice in the 1960s and for much of the 1970s was very congenial to social workers' values and ideological preferences.

Several more recent trends in criminal justice also complement social workers' values and perspectives. Chief among them, perhaps, is the growth of interest in *mediation* and *restorative* justice programs. Mediation programs (also known as alternative dispute resolution and conciliation programs) first began after World War I, in an effort to provide an alternative to formal, adversarial proceedings. Especially since the 1980s, mediation has become an increasingly popular way to bring offenders and victims together to provide them with a constructive way to discuss the impact of the offenders' behavior. Although this is not a realistic option in all instances—for example, crimes involving serious violence where the parties are intensely antagonistic—mediation may be an attractive option when, for example, a victim has lost property as a result of automobile theft or lost money as a result of credit card fraud.

Mediation programs are often based on the concept of restorative justice. Restorative justice is a framework that provides offenders with an opportunity to "right" the "wrongs" for which they are responsible (for example, by making restitution to victims and the community, and by apologizing to victims), and a mechanism to empower victims who wish to confront the offenders responsible for their injuries.

Although such justice system developments—based as they are on concepts such as fairness, justice, empowerment, accountability, and direct communication—complement social workers' values and perspectives, we must acknowledge that they have emerged within a context that is often hostile to social work. Along with enlightened and progressive mediation, restorative justice, and other community-based programs, we find rather harsh and punitive agendas that do not recognize, appreciate, or draw on what social workers have learned about human behavior, misbehavior, and meaningful responses and interventions, where constructive rehabilitation and prevention efforts are balanced with legitimate public safety concerns. Thus, social workers who wish to champion enlightened and progressive prevention and rehabilitation programs must do so alongside colleagues who believe that juvenile offenders should be routinely punished rather than rehabilitated, judges should be guided by strict truth-in-sentencing guidelines that permit little discretion, parole should be eliminated, and prison environments should be stripped of rehabilitation and recreation programs and replaced with punitive, austere settings in order to deter future miscreants.

The challenge for social work is substantial. The painful irony is that social workers now have more to offer than ever before—considering the evolution of the profession's unique knowledge, skills, and values—but they often meet with resistance, suspicion, or outright hostility when they proffer their services in justice settings.

Ideally, social workers would take assertive steps to reclaim their involvement in the justice system. In principle, social workers should be actively involved in all three major phases of the justice system–police, courts, and corrections–and in a variety of roles. More specifically, social workers should reclaim their duties as the following.

Direct Service Providers

There are many opportunities for social workers to assume traditional clinical and direct service functions as, for example, counselors in institutional and community-based settings, and probation and parole officers. However, consistent with social workers' impressive commitment to constructive conflict resolution, social workers should also be active participants in mediation, alternative dispute resolution, restitution, and conciliation programs. Social workers have both the clinical skills to assume these roles and the values and ideological commitment required to be effective. Social work and social workers should be central to the restorative justice movement.

Advocates and Reformers

Social work has always embraced and been committed to social justice issues. Although the profession's track record is somewhat uneven, especially with respect to their recent involvement in and influence on the criminal justice system, social work's history includes a clear and sustained commitment to advocacy and reform. Social workers are trained to identify and confront injustices, through the policy process, protest, and lobbying. Examples of issues that warrant social workers' advocacy and reform efforts include the rights of offenders who have major mental illness, the need for programs designed to facilitate the transition of offenders from institutional to community-based settings, the need to prevent abuse and discrimination in institutional settings, and the legal protection of minors who have been charged and tried in criminal court as adults and sentenced to adult prisons.

Administrators and Supervisors

Social work education programs typically include an administrative track for those students who wish to pursue this career path. Curriculum content ordinarily includes instruction on program planning, budgeting and financial management, grant writing, personnel issues and staff management, employee evaluation, supervision, leadership, staff development, community relations, and organizational dynamics. Such knowledge and skills are invaluable in a wide range of public and private sector criminal justice settings, such as parole and probation offices, residential treatment programs, and counseling centers.

Researchers and Program Evaluators

Throughout the profession's history, social workers have strengthened their understanding of and commitment to research and program evaluation. Criminal justice programs that were once created, designed, and funded based on faith and good will now require in-depth research and evaluation to justify their existence. As the NASW Code of Ethics (1997) states, "social workers should monitor and evaluate policies, the implementation of programs, and practice interventions" (standard 5.02[a]). Every accredited social work education program provides students with at least foundation-level knowledge and skills related to formulating research and evaluation questions, research and evaluation design, sampling methods, data collection techniques, measurement issues (validity and reliability), research and evaluation ethics (especially protection of human subjects), data analysis, and report preparation. These too are invaluable skills in criminal justice settings, particularly in an era where accountability and empirically based evidence of effectiveness are essential.

CONTEXTS FOR ACTION

Social workers have a great deal to contribute in the criminal justice field's three principal contexts: police, the judicial system, and corrections.

Police

Perhaps the least familiar options for social workers are those related to police work. In recent years, many police departments have begun to recognize and appreciate the unique contributions that social workers can make with respect to crisis intervention (for example, assisting with victims and witnesses of child sexual abuse and domestic violence), conducting investigations (for example, interviewing vulnerable victims of serious crimes), assessing individuals' mental health status (especially suicide risk), providing case management services for mentally ill and homeless individuals, making referrals for individuals with drug and alcohol problems, and assisting runaway youths.

A growing number of police departments have added formal victim services programs, many of them staffed by social workers (Knox and Roberts, 2002). Typically, these programs offer crisis intervention services, facilitate police investigations in an effort to avoid re-traumatizing victims, refer victims to service providers in the community (for example, counselors and support groups), and help victims process restitution and compensation claims.

Social workers also have an opportunity to provide clinical services to police officers themselves. Police work is highly stressful, and some officers seek counseling to help them cope with crises and trauma encountered on the job (for example, following a critical incident involving gunfire or the death of a child) and crises in their own personal lives. In some departments social workers provide clinical services to police who are coping with mental health problems, marital or relationship conflict, legal and financial difficulties, and substance abuse. In some instances social workers are on the staff of "in-house" employee assistance programs (EAPs); social workers may also be employed by private agencies with which police departments contract for services.

The Judicial System

Many attorney generals' offices (known in some jurisdictions as the state or district attorney's office) have also drawn on federal or state funding to establish victim and witness assistance programs. These programs, which are ideal settings for social workers, inform crime victims of their rights (for example, with respect to participating in mediation and restitution programs) and the nature of the judicial process (for example, the stages of a prosecution, plea bargaining options, opportunities for victims to testify).

Many judicial systems also employ social workers to screen and refer offenders to various alternative-to-detention and diversion programs (Isenstadt, 1995). In the juvenile justice system, many communities have established ambitious programs designed to place minors who are arrested in their own homes, foster care, or residential programs as an alternative to secure detention prior to adjudication. The goal, especially for status offenders (for example, juveniles charged with ungovernability, curfew violation, and truancy) and minors charged with nonviolent offenses, is to avoid the trauma and harmful consequences of institutional care and incarceration. Also, many courts have established diversion programs designed to provide juveniles and adults with community-based services—such as outpatient counseling programs and residential treatment—that may be more productive than incarceration.

In addition, many public defender offices—the publicly funded offices that provide legal counsel for indigent clients—employ social workers to address the social service needs so often prevalent in the lives of poor defendants. These social workers often conduct assessments and collaborate with their clients' lawyers in an attempt to fashion meaningful alternatives to incarceration that will be acceptable to prosecutors and judges.

The relatively recent advent of drug courts and truancy courts in many jurisdictions has also provided important venues for social workers. These courts operate on the assumption that a significant number of offenders become involved in delinquent and criminal activity as a result of their addiction to alcohol or other drugs or as a result of truancy. The courts typically use a team approach—involving judges, prosecutors, defense attorneys, and social workers—to help offenders and their families receive the help they need. Social workers' knowledge related to addictions, family dynamics, and various intervention models is key to such efforts.

In some jurisdictions, social workers may also participate in competency evaluations. Social workers may work with psychiatrists to facilitate and conduct forensic assessments for individuals who may not be competent to stand trial or who enter a "not guilty by reason of insanity" or "diminished capacity" plea.

Corrections

For decades, social workers have had employment opportunities in juvenile and adult correctional facilities. Typically these positions have included some combination of individual and group counseling duties (general counseling and more specialized counseling related to substance abuse, domestic violence, and sex offenses), crisis intervention services (for example, responding to inmates who have attempted to commit suicide or who have acute psychotic episodes), biopsychosocial assessments upon admission to the institution, and discharge planning for inmates who have been paroled or completed their full sentences. Further, social workers have been employed in a wide range of community-based programs established and operated by departments of corrections, such as halfway houses, transition programs, and electronic-monitoring programs (Butts, 1995).

Large numbers of social workers are also employed as probation or parole officers. Probation officers provide case management and supportive services to individuals who have been offered a suspended sentence or probation as an alternative to incarceration; parole officers provide case management and other social services to offenders who have been granted early release from prison. A growing number of offenders are serving probation or parole on electronic monitoring. Social workers in these positions may provide crisis intervention services and referral for education, vocational, counseling, and substance abuse services. Some state laws also require that a member of the parole board be a social worker or someone with social-service expertise.

Significant numbers of social workers provide community-based services through private social service agencies that have contracts with public corrections agencies. These social workers work closely with corrections staff to provide counseling, outreach and tracking, and school-based prevention programs.

CONCLUSION

For social work to regain its central role in the justice system, prominent organizations in the profession will have to exert genuine and sustained leadership. The Council on Social Work Education, for example, can provide a pivotal service by convening educators interested in the justice system to develop strategies for strengthening education and training on the subject. In addition to offering elective courses on juvenile and criminal justice in departments and schools of social work, educators should develop constructive ways to introduce this content in field placements and in required direct practice, policy, human behavior, and research courses. Using case studies involving individual clients (e.g., effective ways to intervene with individuals convicted of domestic violence, sex offenses, white collar crime, and drug dealing), contemporaneous policy dilemmas (e.g., debates concerning sentencing alternatives, capital punishment, and habitual offender laws), and research challenges (e.g., how to evaluate community-based programs or the effectiveness of a drug court), social work educators can achieve the two-fold goal of helping students cultivate valuable practice, policy, and research skills and learn about the many ways in which social workers can be employed in the justice system. Offering workshops on this topic at CSWE's conferences and publicizing model syllabi, curricula, pedagogical strategies, and field placement opportunities would be major steps.

NASW can also provide critically needed leadership by facilitating meetings at national and statewide conferences among social workers interested in the justice system, sponsoring continuing education on the subject, educating administrators and supervisors in the justice system about social workers' unique and valuable education, and becoming active participants in national and statewide policy debates (e.g., lobbying legislators and administrators, testifying at legislative hearings). There is ample precedent for such activities within NASW with respect to social workers interested in mental health, health care, child welfare, public welfare, and school social work.

Social workers and social justice have been intimate partners throughout the profession's history. During a significant portion of social work's history, preoccupation with justice included both juvenile and criminal justice. It is time for social workers to reconnect with these critically important domains and to contribute its impressive and mature armamentarium of values, knowledge, and skills.

REFERENCES

Barton, W.H. (1995). *Juvenile Corrections.* In R.L. Edwards (Ed.-in-Chief), Encyclopedia of Social Work (19th ed., pp. 1563-1577). Washington, DC: NASW Press.

Berman, S. (1959). *Antisocial Character Disorder: Its Etiology and Relationship to Delinquency.* American Journal of Orthopsychiatry, 29, 612-621.

Bernard, T. (1992). *The Cycle of Juvenile Justice.* New York: Oxford University Press.

Bloch, H.A., & Niederhoffer, A. (1958). *The Gang: A Study in Adolescent Behavior.* New York: Philosophical Library.

Bonczar, R., & Beck, A. (1997). *Lifetime Likelihood of Going to State or Federal Prison.* Washington, DC: U.S. Department of Justice, Office of Justice Programs.

Butts, J.A. (1995). *Community-Based Corrections.* In R.L. Edwards (Ed.-in-Chief), Encyclopedia of Social Work (19th ed., pp. 549-555). Washington, DC: NASW Press.

Cloward, R., & Ohlin, L.E. (1960). *Delinquency and Opportunity.* New York: Free Press.

Cohen, A.K. (1955). *Delinquent Boys: The Culture of the Gang.* Glencoe, IL: Free Press.

Fagan, J., Forst, M., & Vivona, T.S. (1987). *Racial Determinants of the Judicial Transfer Decision Prosecuting Violent Youth in Criminal Court.* Crime and Delinquency, 33, 259-286.

Gibelman, M., & Schervish, P. (1993). *Who We Are: The Social Work Labor Force as Reflected in NASW Membership.* Washington, DC: NASW Press.

Guarino-Ghezzi, S., & Loughran, E.J. (1998). *Balancing Juvenile Justice.* New Brunswick, NJ: Transaction Press.

Hollis, E., & Taylor, A. (Eds.). (1951). *Social Work Education in the United States: The Report of a Study Made for the National Council on Social Work Education.* New York: Columbia University Press.

Hurley, T.D. (1907). *Origin of the Illinois Juvenile Court Law.* Chicago: Visitation and Aid Society.

Iglehart, A.P. (1995). *Criminal Justice: Class, Race, and Gender Issues.* In R.L. Edwards (Ed.-in-Chief), Encyclopedia of Social Work (19th ed., pp. 647-653). Washington, DC: NASW Press.

Isenstadt, P.M. (1995). *Adult Courts.* In R.L. Edwards (Ed.-in-Chief), Encyclopedia of Social Work (19th ed., pp. 68-74). Washington, DC: NASW Press.

Knox, K., & Roberts, A.R. (2002). *Police Social Work.* In A.R. Roberts & G.J. Greene (Eds.), Social Workers' Desk Reference (pp. 668-672). New York: Oxford University Press, 2002.

Krisberg, B., & Austin, J. (1993). *Rethinking Juvenile Justice.* Newbury Park, CA: Sage.

Mann, C.R. (1993). *Unequal Justice: A Question of Color.* Bloomington: Indiana University Press.

Mauer, M. (1997). *Intended and Unintended Consequences of State Racial Disparities in Imprisonment.* Washington, DC: The Sentencing Project.

McNeece, A., & Roberts, A.R. (1997). *Policy and Practice in the Justice System.* Chicago: Nelson-Hall.

Miller, J. (1991). *Last One Over the Wall: The Massachusetts Experiment in Closing Reform Schools.* Columbus: Ohio State University Press.

Miller, J. (1995). *Criminal Justice: Social Work Roles.* In R.L. Edwards (Ed.-in-Chief), Encyclopedia of Social Work (19th ed., pp. 653-659). Washington, DC: NASW Press.

Miller, J. (1996). *Search and Destroy: African American Males in the Criminal Justice System.* New York: Cambridge University Press.

National Association of Social Workers. (1997). *Code of Ethics.* Washington, DC: Author.

National Council of Juvenile and Family Court Judges. (1990). *Minority Youth in the Juvenile Justice System: A Judicial Response.* Juvenile and Family Court Journal, 41 (special issue), 1-71.

Platt, A. (1977). *The Child Savers: The Invention of Delinquency (2nd ed.).* Chicago: University of Chicago Press.

Pope, C.E., & Feyerherm, W. (1993). *Minorities and the Juvenile Justice System: Research Summary.* Washington, DC: U.S. Department of Justice, Office of Juvenile Justice and Delinquency Prevention.

President's Commission on Law Enforcement and the Administration of Justice. (1967). *Task Force Report: Juvenile Delinquency and Youth Crime.* Washington, DC: Government Printing Office.

Quinney, R. (1970). *The Problem of Crime.* New York: Dodd, Mead.

Rapp, C.A. (1998). *The Strengths Model: Case Management with People Suffering from Severe and Persistent Mental Illness.* New York: Oxford University Press.

Reamer, F.G. (2003). *Criminal Lessons: Case Studies and Commentary on Crime and Justice.* New York: Columbia University Press.

Reamer, F.G., & Shireman, C.H. (1981). *Alternatives to the Juvenile Justice System: Their Development and the Current State-of-the-Art.* Juvenile and Family Court Journal, 32, 17-32.

Saleebey, D. (1996). *The Strengths Perspective in Social Work: Extensions and Cautions.* Social Work, 41, 295-305.

Saleebey, D. (Ed.). (1997). *The Strengths Perspective in Social Work Practice (2nd ed.).* New York: Longman.

Sarri, R. (2000). *The Juvenile Justice System in Crisis: Challenges and Opportunities for Social Workers.* In P. Allen-Meares and C. Garvin (Eds.), The Handbook of Social Work Practice (pp. 451-475). Thousand Oaks, CA: Sage.

Shireman, C.H., & Reamer, F.G. (1986). *Rehabilitating Juvenile Justice.* New York: Columbia University Press.

Singer, S. (1996). *Decriminalizing Delinquency: Violent Juvenile Crime and Juvenile Justice Reform.* New York: Cambridge University Press.

Sutherland, E.H., & Cressey, D.R. (1966). *Principles of Criminology (7th ed.).* Philadelphia: J.B. Lippincott.

Tonry, M. (1995). *Malign Neglect: Race, Crime, and the Law.* New York: Oxford University Press.

Tuthill, R.S. (1904). *History of the Children's Court in Chicago.* In S.J. Barrows (Ed.), Children's Courts in the United States. Washington, DC: Government Printing Office.

Wilson, J.Q. (1975). *Thinking About Crime.* New York: Basic Books.

Thirty Years of CURE:
The Struggle Is Its Own Reward

Pauline Sullivan

Charles Sullivan

SUMMARY. The authors describe how, for the past thirty years, they have worked to organize CURE (Citizens United for Rehabilitation of Errants), a prison reform constituency of prisoners and their families. Better rehabilitative opportunities as well as less reliance on incarceration have been the goals of their organization. Beginning in Texas, they have, by trial and error, brought about a community of prison reformers at the local, state, national and international levels. Their organizing principles for this achievement are presented and the reasons for them explained. They conclude that every jail and prison should have an organized monitoring entity of the families of prisoners, and that CURE could be a model. *[Article copies available for a fee from The Haworth Document Delivery Service: 1-800-HAWORTH. E-mail address: <docdelivery@haworthpress.com> Website: <http://www.HaworthPress.com> © 2004 by The Haworth Press, Inc. All rights reserved.]*

Pauline Sullivan, BA, is Administrator of National CURE and has graduate work in special education.

Charles Sullivan, MA, is Executive Director of National CURE and has graduate studies in theology. He has been Adjunct Professor at St. Edwards University in Austin, TX.

Address correspondence to: CURE, National Capital Station, P.O. Box 2310, Washington, DC 20013-2310 (E-mail: cure@curenational.org).

[Haworth co-indexing entry note]: "Thirty Years of CURE: The Struggle Is Its Own Reward." Sullivan, Pauline, and Charles Sullivan. Co-published simultaneously in *Journal of Religion & Spirituality in Social Work* (The Haworth Social Work Practice Press, an imprint of The Haworth Press, Inc.) Vol. 23, No. 1/2, 2004, pp. 233-244; and: *Criminal Justice: Retribution vs. Restoration* (ed: Eleanor Hannon Judah, and Rev. Michael Bryant) The Haworth Social Work Practice Press, an imprint of The Haworth Press, Inc., 2004, pp. 233-244. Single or multiple copies of this article are available for a fee from The Haworth Document Delivery Service [1-800-HAWORTH, 9:00 a.m. - 5:00 p.m. (EST). E-mail address: docdelivery@haworthpress.com].

http://www.haworthpress.com/web/JRSSW
© 2004 by The Haworth Press, Inc. All rights reserved.
Digital Object Identifier: 10.1300/J377v23n01_13

KEYWORDS. Grassroots organizing, prison reform, families of prisoners

Citizens United for Rehabilitation of Errants (CURE) is a national grassroots organization dedicated to reducing crime through reform of the criminal justice system, especially its prisons. The goals of CURE are twofold: (1) to use prisons only for those who have to be in them; and (2) for those who have to be in them, to provide all rehabilitative opportunities they need to "turn their lives around." CURE has chapters in most states and a mailing list of 15,000.

"Don't go up there, it's the men's dorm," came the yell from the bottom of the stairs as Pauline and theologian Rosemary Reuther stopped climbing. When they looked down they saw an elderly woman who seemed to be in charge of this Catholic Worker Hospitality House in New York City. She was in charge! It was 1971 and Dorothy Day had just corrected them. They meekly came down to have tea with Dorothy. By then, Charlie and Mike Cullen, a leader of the Milwaukee 14 who had been recently released from prison for destroying draft records, had parked our van and joined them. We had come to see Dorothy Day after a convention of a grassroots organization that was seeking reform, perhaps revolution, in the Catholic Church. Certainly, with the Vietnam war going on. These were revolutionary times.

To find our place in it, we purchased a '65 Volkswagen van for $800 and left Minneapolis in 1970. All our belongings were in the van, including blankets for sleeping on the floor. We traveled for the next year spending the most time in Texas in the anti-war movement. While visiting friends jailed for civil disobedience, we were shocked by the conditions. In fact, Charlie was arrested and spent a week in the county jail in San Antonio for shouting "too aggressively" at a demonstration protesting these conditions. Later, we were both arrested with thousands in the May Day demonstrations in Washington, DC. "The struggle is its own reward" is how the Texas prisoners ended letters to us. These were the "writ-writers" or "jailhouse lawyers" that risked their lives to file lawsuits.

We asked Dorothy Day what kind of work besides civil disobedience should we be doing. We were surprised that she encouraged us to visit Cuba. Dorothy Day admired Fidel Castro and his achievements in health care and education.

After the visit we drove gain to Washington to lobby against the military draft in Congress. Rosemary Reuther spent an afternoon looking for us in our van on Capitol Hill. A group with religious backgrounds was departing the next day for Havana and they had two cancellations. How different our lives might have been if Rosemary had found us.

At night, we listened to the radio and for almost a week we followed the Attica prison uprising. When the deaths of prisoners and correctional officers were announced, we decided to return to Texas and work long-range on prison reform. We came back to San Antonio and supported ourselves by Pauline's substitute teaching and Charlie driving a taxicab. We began organizing a bus service for families to visit their loved ones in the state prison. Charlie asked then Auxiliary Bishop Patrick Flores, who is now the Archbishop of San Antonio, to be a sponsor of the service, and he eagerly accepted. The American Friends Service Committee also paid us a small stipend. Volunteers mainly from the peace community were recruited as drivers. Thus, CURE really began in San Antonio, on January 2, 1972, at 5 a.m., when the engines of four broken-down buses were started, and their lights turned on. A family member took just about every seat. A community of sisters had spent the day before making hundreds of sandwiches for the riders. We would need this food for the arduous 500-mile round-trip. One mother exclaimed that she hadn't seen her son in ten years while another arrived in her wheelchair and scooted up the bus steps on her rear end.

ESTABLISHING OUR SERVICE

In March of 1972, the city of San Antonio allowed us to use a small rat-infested, abandoned building to sell our bus tickets. It was near the county jail, and we referred those released to agencies that might help them. We called it "The Referral." Later, in December 1972, a dozen of us hurriedly drove to the Capitol in Austin and successfully helped to block the enactment of a new death penalty statute in a special session of the Texas Legislature. The Supreme Court had struck down existent laws and, although we won this time, capital punishment would return with amazing frequency in Texas.

Besides the peace activists, some in the bus service group had family members in prison. And they were emerging as leaders from the bus service. Coming back from Austin, we began to realize that our group needed a name. We decided on CURE (Citizens United for Rehabilitation of Errants). "Citizens" and "rehabilitation" were the right words. Wardens and guards and even prisoners and their families forget that inmates and their loved ones are citizens. Also, surveys showed that the

American people place "rehabilitation" as a top priority for goals of prisons.

We needed a word that began with an "e." Since many families did not want anyone to know they had a loved one in prison, the name "prison" should not be in the name of the organization. So, we got out the dictionary and looked at all the "e's." "Errants," although unusual, seemed to fit. It camouflaged the purpose enough to eliminate this fear. It was also a "cool" name for a "hot" issue. Finally, our Hispanic families liked the name "errants" because in Spanish, it is restorative and nonjudgmental. We all make mistakes!

INMATE GUARDS

In February, we delivered a news release to the media at the Capitol, which announced the formation of our grassroots organization. We also visited legislative offices to seek a sponsor for a prison reform piece of legislation. We wanted this bill introduced in the regular legislative session that began in January and would end in June.

We were discouraged by our negative reception until newly-elected Rep. Joe L. Hernandez, representing San Antonio's poorest district, said he would introduce it. But, what reform should be introduced? We decided a ban on prisoners being used as guards. On the long bus trips, we had heard "horror stories" from families about this so-called "building tender" system. According to the prison officials, these "BTs" were prisoners selected by the administration to do janitorial work, to "tend the buildings." However, they were really used to control the cellblocks. When a warden wanted to stop a prisoner from filing lawsuits, he would ask the BT over his cellblock to threaten, injure or even kill the prisoner. The warden could then say that another prisoner caused the death and that he had nothing to do with it. When wardens were transferred, their "BTs" went with them.

In April, House Bill 1056 by Hernandez passed the House and in May, the Senate. It stated that no inmate could have administrative, disciplinary or supervisory power over another inmate. We naively thought the building tender system would end when the Governor signed the legislation. Ten years would pass before a federal court order forced the prison system to end this brutal and deadly BT system. Two thousand five hundred more correctional officers had to be hired to take the place of these inmate guards. Our bill would be quoted as the reason for this court order.

SERVICE OR ADVOCACY?

In July 1974, we decided to move from San Antonio to Austin. We had accomplished what we set out to do and leadership from the families had developed. Although services and advocacy educate society-at-large, we knew we couldn't do both in the same organization. The prison system liked us when we only ran the bus service. When we advocated banning the building tender system, they saw us "as the enemy." We concluded that CURE would be an advocacy organization, which is what we are today. Although we advocate for services, we do not operate them.

Advocacy is not where the money is because it can be controversial. People and organizations are hesitant to join and commit resources for this reason. Thus, although money is the biggest worry of any grassroots organization, it takes on added stress when you advocate solely and without an actual service program. Because of our commitment to advocacy, we again had to take part-time jobs. Membership fees and donations would be our only source of funding for the next twenty-five years. We are 100% in agreement then and now that CURE must be an advocacy organization!

POLITICS AS ENTERTAINMENT

CURE's criticism of the prison system continued in Austin with our involvement in a legislative study that, for the first time in recent history, addressed fundamental problems with Texas prisons. We also met seasoned legislators that we thought of as "LBJs" on the state level, who introduced us to politics with colorful sayings that we still use, for example, "you have to be on the jury to hang the jury!" "When you are sleeping on the floor, you don't worry about falling out of bed." In other words, take risks because our reform movement is certainly on the floor!

In those days, the House floor was the "best show in town" with the Senate floor a distant second. Many times, eloquence and humor came together to pass or "kill" a bill. The House Speaker was known as "Billy" and some legislators had two first names. Gara LaMarche fresh from New York City to direct the Texas Civil Liberties Union tried to introduce himself to a committee. "Gara" in "translation" was coming out as "Gary." In desperation, Gara said, "Just call me Billy Bob!" The committee nodded in approval.

CHANGES IN LIFESTYLE

Pauline's introduction to the Texas legislative scene occurred one evening when she was visiting members' offices and came across two veteran representatives who had been "tipping a few." They asked her to join them for a drink, which she politely declined. Pauline, not to be deterred, started in on the need for prison reform. After hearing her, they posed a question that we had heard often, but never in such a direct way. "Tell us, little lady, why do you care about those no-good, good-for-nothing, SOB prisoners?"

From this experience, we realized if we were ever going to have any success in prison reform in Texas, we would have to "adjust our marketing strategy." There would be no more arrests for civil disobedience and high profile involvement in the anti-war movement would end for us. In fact, we would not even hold a demonstration. For example, why take a chance on a protest in front of the Governor's mansion when you couldn't control it. Someone could throw a rock and break a window. CURE as sponsor would be finished. Although this seems far-fetched now, we were at the tail end of the sixties and it could have happened. Come to think of it, it could happen today!

We thus joined "the establishment" and became this nice "do-gooder" couple who were properly dressed and who wanted to bring about prison reform. We had become members of the jury to hang the jury! Although some might see us "as part of the problem and not part of the solution," we consider our advocacy another nonviolent means of social change. Lobbying, although under-utilized by activists for social change, is another way besides demonstrations and civil disobedience of "speaking truth to power."

ESTABLISHING OUR ADVOCACY

In 1975, a CURE constitution was written and we had our first state convention. At this gathering, the director of the prison system "walked out" after being publicly questioned by participants. Later, he sent us an apology indicating that he overreacted, but relations with the prison system continued to deteriorate. Besides prison reform, CURE began to focus on jail and probation problems. We aided the creation of the Texas Commission on Jail Standards and the Texas Adult Probation Commission. We also indirectly impacted and influenced community corrections by twice defeating proposals to construct more prisons. These victories were a prelude to *Ruiz v. Estelle*, the longest and most comprehensive prison reform lawsuit in American history. Legendary Federal Judge William Wayne Justice's court orders would reform most of the Texas prison system. CURE helped to facilitate this litigation, now recognized as the prison reform organization in Texas.

In 1978, we opened an office near the Capitol. We also decided not to have a phone at our apartment. Another reason besides money was that we needed to have time and space to "recharge your batteries." There is seemingly always a crisis in prison reform. Another cost-saver was to wear hand-me-down suits from friends and acquaintances. For example, Rep. Joe Hernandez would donate his suits to Charlie. "Whatever Joe wears this legislative session," Charlie would gleefully say, "I will be wearing the next."

THE IMPORTANCE OF PAROLE

We tried to focus on the Parole Board as much as the prison system and were successful in having minorities appointed. Of course, lack of paroles was the problem, and this came to a head when we published "The Maze" which detailed the cumbersome process that parolees went through in 1978. After approval by the Parole Board, the Governor's staff would again review these, rejecting almost one-third. At this time prisons were so overcrowded that prisoners had to sleep in tents set up outside the prisons. "If the Governor would not review the parolees," we hammered away in the media, "there would be no need for the tents." Eventually, Texas voters agreed with us in 1983 and supported a constitutional amendment to remove the Governor from the parole process.

Also in "The Maze" booklet, Pauline had written a question and answer section that encouraged families of prisoners to write their own letters and visit the Parole Board rather than pay an attorney. We were adamant then and still are that an attorney was not needed to be hired to "make parole." Our position came about when we ran The Referral in San Antonio. A mother living in a housing project showed us the letter where an attorney for a thousand dollars had made her son "eligible for parole." We didn't have the heart to tell her that parole eligibility is automatic after one-third of the sentence and that she could have received the same letter from the Parole Board for the cost of a postage stamp. In theory, the Parole Board agreed with us on most of the material in the "Maze" booklet and eventually adopted it as their official informational guide. In fact, another one of our leaders, Minnie Loera, even translated it into Spanish.

Almost twenty years later, in a similar project, CURE developed a resource guide for exoffenders returning to the Washington area. This time, the Federal Bureau of Prisons updated one edition and published it for the BOP staff preparing DC prisoners for reentry.

REPUBLICANS TAKE OVER

In November 1978, Bill Clements in a stunning upset was elected Governor of Texas, the first Republican in history. We presumed that prison reform, which was not very popular with Democrats, would only get worse under Republicans. We were pleasantly surprised. Harry Whittington was appointed to the Prison Board by Governor Clements, and CURE managed to meet with him before his Senate confirmation. Whittington initially was the lone, favorable vote of the nine Prison Board members on reform issues. Eventually, a majority of the other Board members joined him.

Pauline returned to the office from the Capitol one day and announced that a legislator, Rep. Ed Emmett, who wanted to introduce a bill to mandate the prison system to have contact visits, stopped her. A legislator had never stopped us and when we looked up the background of this particular one, we couldn't believe our eyes. He was a Republican! "Out of the blue," Rep. Ed Emmett later explained that he was invited to speak at the high school graduation at one of the prisons. After his speech, when he "was working the crowd," he came across a little boy about four years old in the arms of his prisoner father. Both were crying.

Rep. Emmett thought at first this was because of the father's graduation. "No," the dad said, "this is the first time that I have ever touched my son." He explained that his son had been born after he was imprisoned. Although they had visited, there were no contact visits except for rare occasions like graduations. At that time, Rep. Emmett had a four-year-old son and could not imagine not being able to touch and hold his son. Legislation was introduced in the next session of the Legislature and we organized families "to hit the right political note" during legislative hearings on Emmett's bill. This was extremely helpful in the passage of the bill.

We had already left for Washington when contact visits became a reality in the prisons. Later, when Charlie returned to one of the prison units and saw the outside contact visiting settings, he was moved to tears.

Besides helping to "soften" up the Texas legislature to support contact visits, CURE also was instrumental in passing another pro-family initiative, a five-day furlough program. After Ruiz, we made a deliberate decision to move from confrontation approaches to cooperative strategies that encouraged the state to comply with the court order and not support appeal of it. In 1981, this resulted in a token legislative response to the court order. For example, the Governor after two vetoes finally signed the bill to remove automatic restrictions on felons for sixty occupational licenses.

In the 1983 Session, however, our encouraging attitude played a role in the Legislature having its most productive prison reform session in history. Millions for prison expansion were shifted to community corrections. In 1984 our relationship with the prison system stopped its downward spiral when the new director spoke at our convention. The result of this relationship was the passage of the ex-felon legislation, including the last issue in Ruiz. Overcrowding was settled.

EXPANDING NATIONALLY

In August 1985, we rented a U-haul truck, packed our belongings and drove to Washington. For some time, we had been thinking of trying to expand CURE. Although there were other national prison organizations, there was not one that focused on prisoners and their families. Pauline had made clear that she would not move unless we had $10,000 in the bank. Before leaving, we had a fund-raiser that netted $12,000.

As we did in Texas 15 years before in the Texas legislature, Charlie spend hours "walking the halls," this time in Congress looking for support. One day, tired and discouraged, he "caught" Congressman, John Conyers, Jr. of Detroit, the Chairman of the Criminal Justice Subcommittee, after a hearing. Charlie gave him a "30 second explanation" of CURE in the hallway. He was startled when Congressman Conyers not only was impressed, but also asked him "if he had the time" would he come with him to his office and give him a fuller explanation? As Rep. Joe Hernandez did for Texas CURE in 1973, Congressman Conyers did for National CURE in 1987. He put us "on the map!"

Congressman Conyers was the keynote speaker at our first national convention that was held in June. At this event, he announced then that he and Charlie would start Michigan-CURE in his congressional office in Detroit.

Our first issue in Congress was a repeat of our experience in Texas too. This time working with a coalition, we failed again in stopping the enactment of the death penalty. We also "played defense" in regard to massive prison expansion and were not successful. Like Texas, Congress seemed to be determined to solve the crime problem by executing people and building prisons. We did, however, amend the Women, Infants and Children Program (WIC) to include pregnant prisoners and increasing the Prison Industry Enhancement Program (PIE) to all states. Although opposed to private prisons, CURE strongly supports the privatization of prison industries, which means good jobs for good wages. Besides family support and employable skills, education is also a key element for rehabilitation. We helped in creation of an Office of Correctional Education within the U.S. Department of Education.

Finally, other state chapters were established, and periodic conferences on chapter leader development were conducted. In 1991, issue chapters were organized. These chapters would be national in membership and would focus on specific issues such as treatment for sex offenders and organizing families with loved ones on death row.

COULD THINGS GET ANY WORSE?

Since coming to Washington in the mid-eighties, we had suffered setbacks under Republican Presidents and naively longed for a Democrat in the White House. Thus, we were totally unprepared for the Clinton/Reno "law and order" agenda expressed in the 1994 Crime Bill. Capital punishment was added to fifty more crimes and millions were authorized to build prisons. Pell Grants for prisoners were terminated.

In 1995, our reforms in the Crime Bill for incarcerated veterans and correctional officer training were also eliminated, and the Family Unity Demonstration Project, a program to allow nonviolent offenders to serve their sentences with their small children, was never funded. In 1996, prisoners were severely limited in the filing of lawsuits. Our only wins were an Office of Correctional Job Training and Placement within the U.S. Department of Justice and the creation of Specter Grants, which provided a smaller replacement for Pell Grants. Within CURE this depressing picture seemed to be mirrored. From 1997-2000, six CURE leaders died. Two died unexpectedly and one was executed by the state of Texas.

SIGNIFICANT PROGRESS

Like the Phoenix and in the spirit of the paschal mystery of Christianity, we seemed to build from these ashes. Equitable Telephone Charges, CURE's highly successful national campaign to reduce the costs of inmate phones, was launched. Coordinated by National CURE Chairperson Kay Perry, the focus is on the families of prisoners who had to pay these exorbitant costs since prisoners could only call collect. This Campaign substantially expanded the efforts of our pro-bono attorneys who had been making this argument for price reduction before the Federal Communications Commission.

The ETC Campaign was followed by For Whom the Bells Toll, an initiative to have religious organizations toll their bells whenever there is an execution. Where there is no bell tower, people are encouraged to hang a black drape outside the building or tie black ribbons on poles. Longtime CURE leader Sister Dorothy Briggs O.P. leads this Campaign.

Also, CURE helped to facilitate the U.S. Catholic Bishops Criminal Justice Statement. In fact, CURE is specifically mentioned on page 3 of the 40-page document, and most of the pictures used in the booklet were taken by our photographer, Alan Pogue. Since CURE's beginning, Alan has volunteered to photograph our events. His documentary photography on prisons and other social issues has now been recognized internationally.

Finally, the Clinton Administration began to provide leadership in prison reform. For example, Attorney General Janet Reno was able to have 100 million dollars appropriated to aid the re-entry efforts of serious and violent offenders. CURE recently has been involved in four far-reaching reforms by Congress:

1. All deaths in custody would have to be reported to the U.S. Department of Justice and annual statistics compiled on them. This legislation was similar to the bill we passed in Texas;
2. The section in the U.S. Department of Justice that sues prisons and jails for unconstitutional conditions received its first staff increase in its twenty year history;
3. The U.S. Department of Veterans' Affairs was mandated to assist incarcerated veterans with reentry;
4. Mental health courts were created in which nonviolent mentally ill offenders will be diverted from going to jail if they seek treatment.

Further, in 2001, CURE's International Conference on Human Rights and Prison Reform in New York City was a success even though it was held three weeks after the tragic events of September 11th. Two hundred twenty-five participants from twenty-four countries attended. These countries were asked to introduce a resolution in the UN that would "make real" the principle of universal suffrage in regard to prisoners. We will be going to Geneva, Switzerland, to continue to lobby for the introduction of this resolution. Over the years, mobilizing voting by families of prisoners, former prisoners and now even prisoners has been CURE's top priority to solve the problems of prisons.

THE FUTURE

We are both in our sixties and struggling with our exit strategy. We would like to establish an endowment in order that the new staff of National CURE would have a "cushion" to operate. Should we follow up on our international conference and expand internationally? We have tried and many times succeeded in providing "a place at the table" for prisoners and their loved ones when correctional policy decisions are made. Governors, legislators, prison directors and wardens have had to at least consider formal positions by an organized, totally independent constituency of volunteers. Whether CURE is the name of this type of prisoner consumer movement/organization remains to be seen. And, when you get right down to it, the name is really not that important. But, a organization like CURE should be keeping an eye on every prison and jail in the world!

Index

BOOK ORDER FORM!

Order a copy of this book with this form or online at:
http://www.haworthpress.com/store/product.asp?sku=5054

Criminal Justice
Retribution vs. Restoration

___ in softbound at $29.95 (ISBN: 0-7890-0081-4)
___ in hardbound at $39.95 (ISBN: 0-7890-0061-X)

COST OF BOOKS _____	❑ **BILL ME LATER:**
	Bill-me option is good on US/Canada/ Mexico orders only; not good to jobbers, wholesalers, or subscription agencies.
POSTAGE & HANDLING _____	
US: $4.00 for first book & $1.50 for each additional book	❑ **Signature** _____
Outside US: $5.00 for first book & $2.00 for each additional book.	❑ **Payment Enclosed: $** _____
SUBTOTAL _____	❑ **PLEASE CHARGE TO MY CREDIT CARD:**
In Canada: add 7% GST. _____	❑ Visa ❑ MasterCard ❑ AmEx ❑ Discover
STATE TAX _____	❑ Diner's Club ❑ Eurocard ❑ JCB
CA, IL, IN, MN, NY, OH & SD residents please add appropriate local sales tax.	**Account #** _____
FINAL TOTAL _____	**Exp Date** _____
If paying in Canadian funds, convert using the current exchange rate. UNESCO coupons welcome.	**Signature** _____
	(Prices in US dollars and subject to change without notice.)

PLEASE PRINT ALL INFORMATION OR ATTACH YOUR BUSINESS CARD

Name

Address

City   State/Province   Zip/Postal Code

Country

Tel   Fax

E-Mail

May we use your e-mail address for confirmations and other types of information? ❑ Yes ❑ No We appreciate receiving your e-mail address. Haworth would like to e-mail special discount offers to you, as a preferred customer. **We will never share, rent, or exchange your e-mail address.** We regard such actions as an invasion of your privacy.

Order From Your **Local Bookstore** or Directly From
The Haworth Press, Inc. 10 Alice Street, Binghamton, New York 13904-1580 • USA
Call Our toll-free number (1-800-429-6784) / Outside US/Canada: (607) 722-5857
Fax: 1-800-895-0582 / Outside US/Canada: (607) 771-0012
E-mail your order to us: orders@haworthpress.com

For orders outside US and Canada, you may wish to order through your local
sales representative, distributor, or bookseller.
For information, see http://haworthpress.com/distributors

(Discounts are available for individual orders in US and Canada only, not booksellers/distributors.)

Please photocopy this form for your personal use.
www.HaworthPress.com

BOF04